BRADY

SUCCESS! in ACLS

Tips and Tricks for Passing the ACLS Course

Shaun Fix, EMT-P

Kathleen Lezon, RN

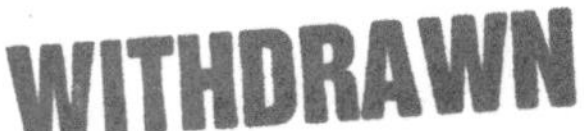

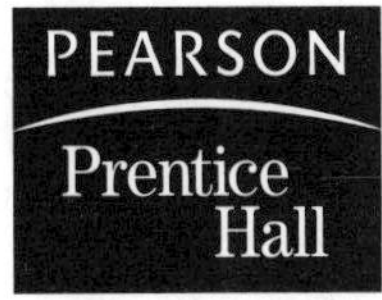

Upper Saddle River, New Jersey 07458

Publisher: Julie Levin Alexander
Publisher's Assistant: Regina Bruno
Senior Acquisitions Editor: Stephen Smith
Associate Editor: Monica Moosang
Editorial Assistant: Patricia Linard
Director of Marketing: Karen Allman
Executive Marketing Manager: Katrin Beacom
Marketing Coordinator: Michael Sirinides
Marketing Assistant: Wayne Celia, Jr.
Managing Production Editor: Patrick Walsh
Production Liaison: Julie Li
Production Editor: Karen Fortgang, bookworks
Manufacturing Manager: Ilene Sanford
Manufacturing Buyer: Pat Brown
Senior Design Coordinator: Christopher Weigand
Composition: Techbooks
Printing and Binding: Bind Rite Graphics
Cover Printer: Coral Graphics

Notice on Gender Usage

The English language has historically given preference to the male gender. Among many words, the pronouns "he" and "his" are commonly used to describe both genders. Society evolves faster than language, and the male pronouns still predominate our speech. Therefore, male pronouns are used to describe both males and females solely for the purpose of brevity. This is not intended to offend any readers.

Pearson Education LTD.
Pearson Education Singapore, Pte. Ltd
Pearson Education, Canada, Ltd
Pearson Education–Japan
Pearson Education Australia PTY, Limited
Pearson Education North Asia Ltd
Pearson Educación de Mexico, S.A. de C.V.
Pearson Education Malaysia, Pte. Ltd

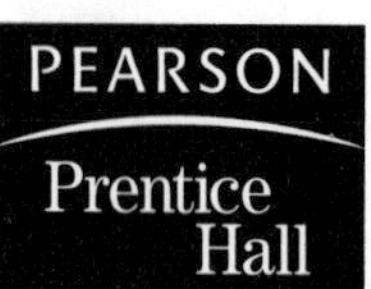

10 9 8 7 6 5 4 3 2 1
ISBN: 0-13-117621-8

About the Authors

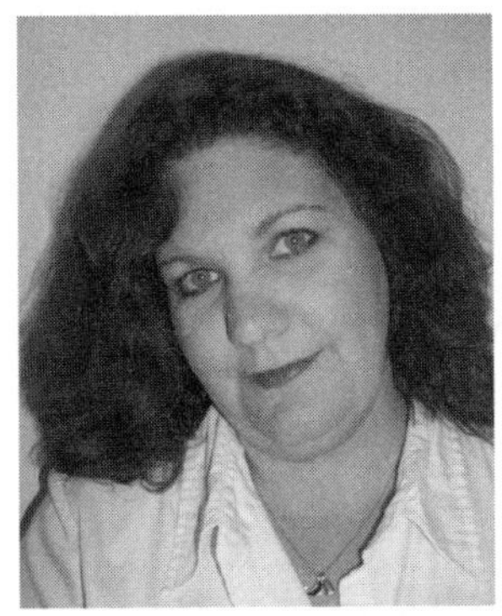

Kathy Lezon, involved in nursing clinical and education arenas since 1986, received her nursing education at St. Vincent Hospital School of Nursing in Worcester, Massachusetts. During her career as a critical care nurse, nurse manager, wound care specialist, and clinical educator, Kathy has earned certifications in wound care, neuroscience nursing, and critical care nursing as well as a certificate in Human Resource Development and Training from Florida Atlantic University. Kathy has published articles in several nursing journals and contributed a chapter to a book on Nursing Management. In the classroom teaching ACLS weekly, Kathy is known for her ability to teach complex concepts in a relaxed, understandable manner. President of Healthcare Education Resources, Inc., and Director of Operations of Emergency Medical Consultants, Inc., Kathy is active in emergency cardiac care training and community activities on the Treasure Coast of Florida.

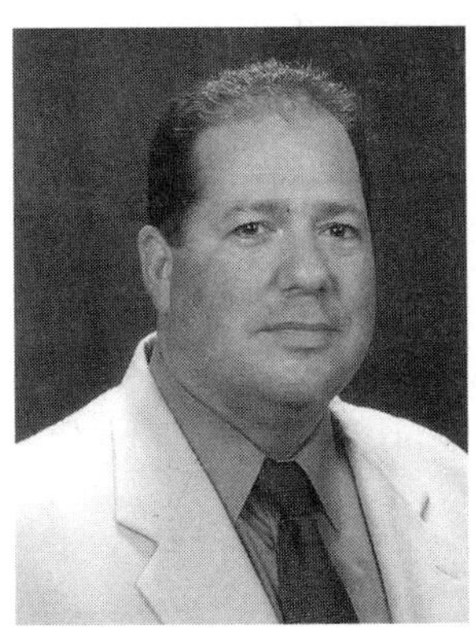

Shaun Fix has been practicing and teaching in the hospital and prehospital field since 1983. He holds a degree in EMS management, is an adjunct faculty member at several colleges, and as a company officer oversees EMS for Boca Raton Fire Rescue Services in South Florida. Since 1988 Shaun has also been the president of Emergency Medical Consultants, Inc., a corporation that provides continuing education for over 15,000 medical professionals annually. Shaun has been involved in course design and presentation of the ACLS material for more than 20 years and continues to present ACLS programs regularly to medical professionals of all levels of expertise.

Reviewers

Brenda M. Beasley, RN, BS, EMT-P
Chair, Allied Health Dept.
Calhoun College
Decatur, AL

Harvey Conner, AS, NREMT-P
EMS Programs
Oklahoma City Community College
Oklahoma City, OK

Robert Hawkes
Program Director, EMS Department
Southern Maine Technical College
South Portland, ME

Sean Kivlehan, EMT-P
EMS Instructor
New York Presbyterian Hospital
New York, NY

John Lewis, MEd., NREMT-P
Paramedic Program Director
Brigham Young University
Rexburg, ID

Shelby L. Louden, B.Sc., EMT-P; EMSI
Partner, Education Associates
Cincinnati, OH

Kenneth Navarro
CE Coordinator
University of Texas Southwestern
Dallas, TX

Scott R. Snyder BS, NREMT-P
Folsom, CA

Jarrod Taylor, NREMT-P, RN, BSN
Calhoun Community College
Decatur, AL

Jim Williams, NR/CCEMT-P, RN
Field Operations Manager
Medical Center at Bowling Green
Emergency Medical Services
Bowling Green, KY

Contents

Introduction

Thank you for choosing Success! in *ACLS: Tips and Tricks for Passing the ACLS Course* to help you prepare for your ACLS class. We hope that this study guide, along with your ACLS textbook, effective instruction, and plenty of preparation on your part, will turn your ACLS experience into a rewarding and beneficial one.

With so much information to piece together in a short ACLS class, here are some tips on how to approach the task:

1. Start early! Schedule your attendance at an ACLS provider course and begin studying as far in advance as possible. This will allow you time to prepare and to minimize the chance that you'll be doing last-minute cramming.
2. Read the book! This guide is meant to be a supplement to whatever textbook is required by your course's sanctioning agency. Groups of scientific and educational experts have collaborated to present to you the most up-to-date resuscitation guidelines available.
3. Plan on learning, not just memorizing! Whether you are taking ACLS for the first or the tenth time, if you understand the "why's" behind recommendations and treatments, you are more likely to make the correct decision when working through scenarios or encountering a real-life clinical situation.
4. Ask questions! If something in your course is not clear, utilize the experts that have been assigned to teach you. Chances are, if you have a question about a particular topic, someone else in the room is wondering about the same thing.
5. Remember comfort! It's hard to learn if you're tired or hungry or hot or cold. Get plenty of rest before your course, eat breakfast and make plans for a healthy lunch, and dress appropriately for the classroom

setting, where you may experience temperature changes throughout the day. (Think "layers"!)

6. Relax! Try to have fun. Remember, that which is learned with laughter is truly learned.

As the subtitle implies, tips and tricks for passing the ACLS course is our focus with this manual. The text intentionally utilizes generic terminology and attempts to simplify sometimes complex concepts relating to ACLS. The generic terminology makes this manual applicable to all ACLS programs from any sanctioning body and for any level provider. Our goal is to give you an *understanding* of cardiac care management rather than having you merely memorize some treatment guidelines; thus you will be able to provide care for a patient and his specific condition rather than simply monitoring the patient. A true learning experience is gained when the provider can actually relate these concepts to everyday patient care.

The text is broken into segments that highlight the mandatory areas of ACLS with an emphasis on "Keeping it simple" and providing the "Need to know" information. Information is presented in a way that relates to its clinical significance and priority in true patient management.

The sections include assessment and treatment skills such as CPR, airway management, and ECG recognition. The manual then discusses pharmacology and cardiac conditions including acute coronary syndromes, stroke, and the complications associated with these illnesses. Finally, the "Putting it all together" portion incorporates the assessment and treatment sections to provide a simplified version of the nationally recognized patient management algorithms. Plenty of practice questions help to reinforce the information throughout the program.

This text is designed to help you understand the concepts of ACLS and how it applies to actual patient care in the ACLS course as well as in actual practice. We realize it is impossible to teach psychomotor skills such as *how* to intubate or start an IV, thus our goal is to present a global approach to patient cases rather than focus on a specific skill that may or may not be part of your clinical practice.

Reviewing the in-depth information in your ACLS course text, utilizing this preparatory material, and answering the review questions will yield a truly stress-free ACLS program and enhance your understanding of managing cardiac patients.

Guidelines: 2005 Changes

In late 2005, the most recent guidelines for Cardiopulmonary Resuscitation and Emergency Cardiac Care were published in *Circulation* (Vol. 112, Issue 24 Supplement; December 13, 2005). These recommendations have changed the content of resuscitation courses from all agencies. If you are taking ACLS for the first time, then don't worry—you don't have information to "unlearn." If you are a repeat ACLS participant, then the following summary of the changes may assist you in remembering what's new.

RESPIRATORY EMERGENCIES

- If cervical spine injury is suspected, use the jaw thrust to open the airway. If the jaw thrust does not open the airway, use the head tilt–chin lift maneuver.
- Each breath given during CPR should be delivered over 1 second, providing enough volume to produce visible chest rise. Deliver these short breaths regardless of method of delivery (mouth-to-mouth, mouth-to-mask, bag-valve-mask, via advanced airway, and with or without oxygen).
- An advanced airway may not be an immediate priority. Rescuers should weigh the need for airway insertion against the need for compression.
- Devices such as an LMA or a Combitube may be an acceptable substitute for the endotracheal tube, depending on rescuers, patient, and setting.
- Confirmation procedures such as CO_2 detection should be considered primary, and should accompany clinical assessment following advanced airway placement.
- Rescue breathing for adults with an advanced airway in place during CPR should be delivered at a rate of 8–10 breaths per minute, as part of "asynchronous" delivery of compressions and ventilations.

- When a choking victim becomes unconscious, rescuers should activate the emergency response process and begin CPR beginning with opening the airway, checking in the mouth for a visible object before each breath is given, and sweeping the mouth to remove an object if one is seen.

VENTRICULAR FIBRILLATION TREATED WITH CPR AND AN AED

- Be sure to allow for complete chest wall recoil during compressions.
- Utilize a 30:2 compression to ventilation ratio.
- Do not interrupt chest compressions to apply AED pads.
- Deliver one shock with the AED and follow immediately with CPR, beginning with compressions. Note: AEDs issued before 2006 may need to be updated to follow this sequence.

VENTRICULAR FIBRILLATION, PULSELESS VENTRICULAR TACHYCARDIA

- Same CPR and defibrillation guidelines as V-fib with CPR and AED.
- For manual defibrillation: 1 shock with the following energy:
  360 J monophasic waveform
  150–200 J biphasic truncated exponential waveform
  120 J biphasic rectilinear waveform
  200 J if not sure what kind of biphasic waveform
  Subsequent shocks: 1 shock at same energy or higher
- Sequence interventions CPR-Shock-CPR-Shock, with medications given during CPR Rhythm check following shock will occur after 2 minutes of CPR is completed.
- Vasopressor medications: Epinephrine 1 mg q 3–5 min. Vasopressin 40 IU may be used as an alternative to the first or second dose of epinephrine. Vasopressin is used only once. Epinephrine added in 3–5 minutes if patient remains pulseless.
- Antiarrhythmic medications: Amiodarone 300 mg considered best choice. If Amiodarone is not available, Lidocaine may be used.

ANY CARDIAC ARREST

- If a victim of any age has a sudden witnessed collapse, the arrest is likely to be cardiac in nature, so lone healthcare providers should immediately call for help, retrieve the AED or defibrillator, and defibrillate as soon as possible.
- If a victim of any age has a likely asphyxial arrest, the lone healthcare provider should provide about 2 minutes of CPR before leaving the victim to call for help and get the AED.
- Organize interventions to minimize interruptions in compressions.

PULSELESS ELECTRICAL ACTIVITY

- Vasopressor medications: Epinephrine 1 mg q 3–5 min. Vasopressin 40 IU may be used as an alternative to the first or second dose of epinephrine. Vasopressin is used only once. Epinephrine added in 3–5 minutes if patient remains pulseless.
- Hypoglycemia and trauma added to the list of Hs and Ts to consider when looking for reversible causes of arrest.

ASYSTOLE

- Pacing no longer recommended as an intervention for patients in asystole.
- Vasopressor medications: Epinephrine 1 mg q 3–5 min. Vasopressin 40 IU may be used as an alternative to the first or second dose of epinephrine. Vasopressin is used only once. Epinephrine added in 3–5 minutes if patient remains pulseless.

ACUTE CORONARY SYNDROMES

- Early use of aspirin is emphasized by the recommendation that EMS dispatcher may instruct callers about chest pain to chew aspirin prior to the arrival of EMS.
- Clopidogrel (Plavix) has been added to the algorithm.

SYMPTOMATIC BRADYCARDIA

- The Atropine dose has been changed to 0.5 mg IV rather than 0.5–1.0 mg.

UNSTABLE TACHYCARDIA

- Treatment recommendations for unstable tachycardia, whether wide or narrow complex, are the same. Emphasis is on determining if the patient is showing signs of rate-related hemodynamic compromise, and if so, preparing for synchronized cardioversion.
- Energy for cardioversion:
  Ventricular tach, atrial fibrillation: 100–200 J monophasic
  100–120 J biphasic
  Atrial flutter and other SVTs: 50–100 monophasic
  100–120 biphasic
  Subsequent shocks at higher doses
- Polymorphic VT—do not synchronize, 360 J monophasic
  150–200 J biphasic truncated
  120 J biphasic rectilinear
  Subsequent doses same or higher energy

- Increased emphasis on finding and treating the cause of dysrhythmias. Hs and Ts found in arrest algorithms included in this algorithm.

STABLE TACHYCARDIA

- Classify stable tachycardias as wide versus narrow and regular versus irregular.

CHAPTER 1

The Basics

Rules for Keeping Yourself Out of Trouble…in ACLS and in Life!

Be Nice	"Good professionals get into trouble, bad professionals get into trouble. . . . Nice professionals don't get into as much trouble."
Rule 1	Treat the patient, not the monitor. (Check pulses and vital signs.)
Rule 2	Always remember Rule 1.
Rule 3	If you ARE treating the patient for an arrhythmia—always treat in this order: *Rate*, then *rhythm*, then *blood pressure*.

ACLS Course Objectives

There are several organizations that present curricula for Advanced Cardiac Life Support, but no matter who awards your certification, course objectives are pretty similar. By the time you successfully complete an ACLS course, you should be able to:

1. Describe patient situations that may require the administration of emergency cardiac care.
2. Conduct primary and secondary ABCD survey.
3. Manage, within the scope of your practice, each of the ACLS cases using the ACLS algorithms.

4. Demonstrate, within the scope of your practice, the airway management, cardioversion, defibrillation, and pacing skills included in the ACLS patient management guidelines.
5. Manage the first few minutes of a ventricular fibrillation/pulseless ventricular tachycardia arrest.

The tools that will help you meet these objectives include:

1. The ability to perform basic life support
2. The ability to recognize basic arrhythmias
3. An understanding of ACLS pharmacology
4. Proficient use of the cardiac monitor/defibrillator/pacer equipment
5. An understanding of the patient assessment and reassessment required
6. Mastery of the sequence of each ACLS algorithm

For Perfusing Patients (People with Pulses)

Start with:

Begin with the basics of all patient care:

Assess and maintain **A**irway, **B**reathing, and **C**irculation.

Evaluates the patient's symptoms and related history. Begin a physical exam.

Things to do:

Administer oxygen.

Assess and monitor vital and diagnostic signs: respirations, pulse, B/P, pulse oximetry, monitor EKG rhythm.

Establish vascular access.

Things to order:

12-lead ECG

Blood work, specifically cardiac enzymes

Chest X-ray

PRIMARY A B C D

A Airway—open it by placing the patient in the sniffing position.

B Breathing—assess breathing for less than 10 seconds. If breathing is absent, provide 2 breaths over 1 second each, then continue once approximately every 8–10 seconds.

C Circulation—evaluate for signs of a pulse. If pulse is absent, begin and maintain compressions at 100/minute.

D Defibrillator—bring and attach a monitor/defibrillator to the patient. Shock when appropriate.

SECONDARY A B C D

A Advanced airway procedures. Reserved for those skilled at these procedures (tracheal, esophageal, or laryngeal tube).

B Breathing assessed, assured, and secured. Be sure whichever tube is placed is causing chest rise, apply supplemental O_2, then secure the device.

C Circulatory interventions. Establish or confirm vascular access and begin cardiac pharmacology. *Hint:* In cardiac arrest the first medication is always a vasopressor such as epinephrine or vasopressin. Then continue epinephrine each 3-5 minutes.

D Differential diagnosis. Search for reversible causes if management according to the standard flow chart is not yielding a successful resuscitation.

Potential Reversible Causes of Cardiac Arrest

Hypovolemia	**T**ablets or **T**oxins
Hypoxia	**T**amponade, cardiac
Hydrogen ion-acidosis	**T**ension pneumothorax
Hyper/hypokalemia	**T**hrombosis-coronary
Hypothermia	**T**hrombosis-pulmonary
Hypoglycemia	**T**rauma
	Too fast or too slow

Skills Review

THE ABCs OF CPR

Determine unresponsiveness—stimulate and shout, "Are you okay?"
If no response—"Help! / call 911."

A = Airway—open the airway with head tilt/chin lift.

B = Breathing—look, listen, and feel; if no, give 2 breaths.

C = Circulation—check for definite pulse in < 10 seconds.

D = Defibrillate if appropriate.

CPR Reference

	Adults (< puberty)	**2 Person**	**Children (1–puberty)**	**Infants (< 1 yr)**
Rescue breathing, Victim definitely has a pulse	10–12 breaths/min; recheck pulse every 2 min	N/A	12–20 breaths/min; recheck pulse every 2 min	12–20 breaths/min; recheck pulse every 2 min
No pulse (or pulse <60 in infant or child with poor perfusion)—compression landmark:	Middle of the chest, between the nipples	Middle of the chest, between the nipples	Middle of the chest, between the nipples	1 finger below nipple line
Compressions are performed with:	Heel of 2 hands	Heel of 2 hands	Heel of 1 or 2 hands	2 fingers OR 2 thumbs when using encircling hands technique
Rate of compressions per minute	100	100	100	at least 100
Compression depth:	1½–2 inches	1½–2 inches	⅓ to ½ depth of chest	⅓–½ depth of chest
Ratio of compressions to breaths:	30:2 Change compressors and reevaluate every 2 min	30:2 Change compressors and reevaluate every 2 min	30:2 15:2 if 2 rescuers Change compressors and reevaluate every 2 min	30:2 15:2 if 2 rescuers Change compressors and reevaluate every 2 min

Foreign Body Airway Obstruction

If not rapidly removed call Emergency Medical Service

Conscious

Adult	**Child**	**Infant**
Abdominal thrusts	Abdominal thrusts (Heimlich maneuver)	5 back blows/ 5 chest thrusts

Unconscious

Adult	Child	Infant
Call EMS. Begin ABCs of CPR. Before giving breaths, look in mouth for foreign body. Use finger sweep to remove object if it is seen. Repeat cycles of CPR until EMS arrives.	Begin CPR. If second rescuer is present, send them to call 911; otherwise, call EMS after 2 minutes of CPR. Before giving breaths, look in mouth for foreign body. Use finger sweep to remove object if it is seen. Repeat cycles of CPR until EMS arrives.	Begin CPR. If second rescuer is present, send them to call 911; otherwise, call EMS after 2 minutes of CPR. Before giving breaths, look in mouth for foreign body. Use finger sweep to remove object if it is seen. Repeat cycles of CPR until EMS arrives.

CHAPTER 2

Airway Management

Oxygen Administration and Airway Management

DETERMINE THE NEED

Patients experiencing cardiovascular emergencies should receive oxygen by some means. Evaluate the patient for any of the following: chest discomfort, dyspnea, neurological symptoms, general weakness, altered mentation, or any signs of hypoxia. Remember pulse oximetery is an excellent evaluation tool, but not the only factor in evaluating oxygen requirements. Clinical presentation should take precedence over reading a monitor. Treat the patient, not merely the monitoring devices.

Quick Tip

Understanding Pulse Oximetry

The "pulse ox" device measures the saturation of the hemoglobin molecule. The provider should remember that a pulse oximetry level of 90% is only equal to an arterial blood gas PaO_2 of 60 torr while the normal blood gas value is 80–100 torr.

Pulse ox of 95–100%—normal. Consider nasal cannula for cardiac patients.

Pulse ox of 90–95%—mild to moderate hypoxia. Use nasal cannula or face mask.

Pulse ox of 85–90%—moderate to severe hypoxia. Use nonrebreather or BVM assist.

Pulse ox below 85%—severe hypoxia. Assist ventilations, consider advanced tubes.

OXYGEN ADMINISTRATION

For Spontaneously Breathing Patients, Consider the Following:

Nasal cannula @ 1–6 lpm (24–44%) for minimally distressed stable patients (Figure 2-1a).

Simple face mask @ 6–10 lpm (35–60%) for moderately distressed patients.

Nonrebreather mask @ 10–15 lpm (95–100%) for signs of more significant distress (Figure 2-1b).

Venturi mask @ 4–12 lpm (24–50%) for patients who require more precise O_2 levels.

Figure 2-1 (A) Nasal cannula (B) Nonrebreather mask

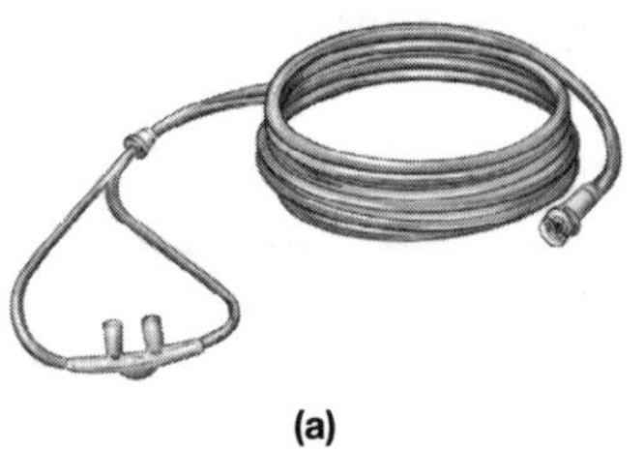

(a)

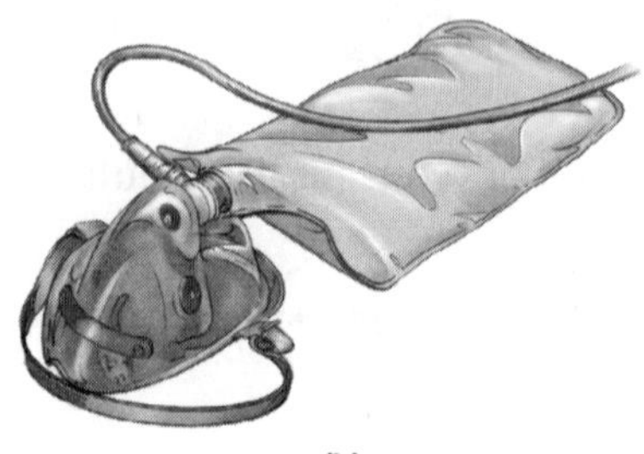

(b)

Please note: The following psychomotor skills are discussed globally and generically regarding technique. An ACLS course does not provide licensure or certification to perform a specific skill. Practitioners who are authorized to perform such skills in their professional role must follow the guidelines and procedures set forth by their experience, clinical setting, or local policy.

Consider the following.

Positive Pressure Ventilation Via Bag Valve Mask Technique

Bag valve mask ventilation with oxygen reservoir and supplemental oxygen (10–15 lpm) can provide nearly 100% oxygen to the patient when used appropriately. Assisted bag valve mask ventilations are indicated for patients in respiratory arrest, or in severe respiratory compromise with either inadequate tidal volumes or oxygen levels.

Using the bag valve mask (Figure 2-2):

1. Maintain an open airway by placing the patient in the sniffing position using the head tilt-chin lift or, if spinal injury is suspected, use the modified jaw thrust.
2. Position yourself at the patient's head and seal the mask from the bridge of nose to the mandible. Position your hands in the "E and C" positions. This can be done by one person but is more effective with two rescuers (one to secure the mask, the other to ventilate).
3. Ventilate slowly (over 1 second) only enough to achieve chest rise. The appropriate rate is approximately 10 breaths per minute (about every 6 seconds). An assistant can provide gentle cricoid pressure by pushing down on the larynx to reduce gastric filling and vomiting potential during bag valve mask ventilations.
4. *Note:* Bag mask ventilations ALWAYS take precedence over intubation and other

Figure 2-2a Head tilt-chin lift

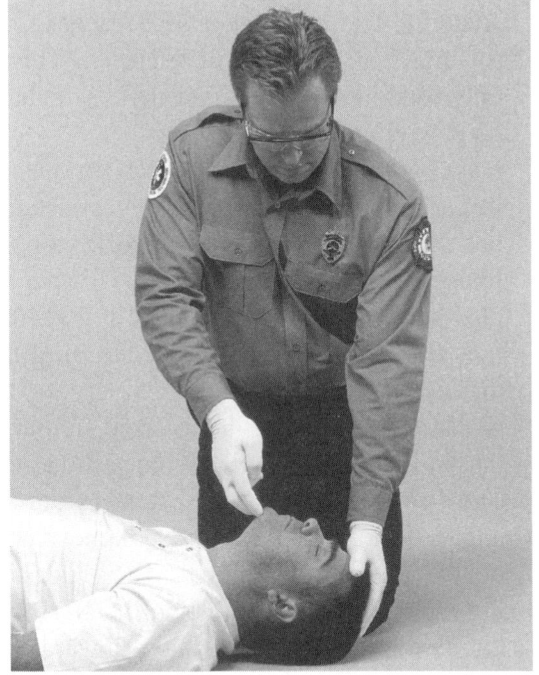
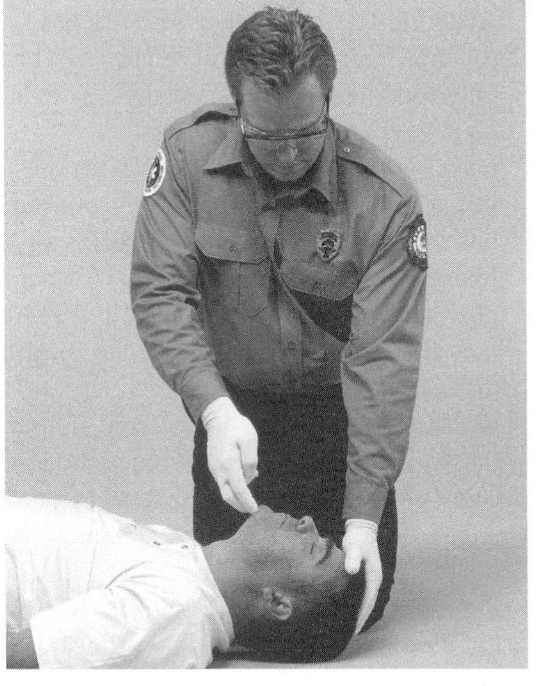

Figure 2-2b Modified jaw thrust

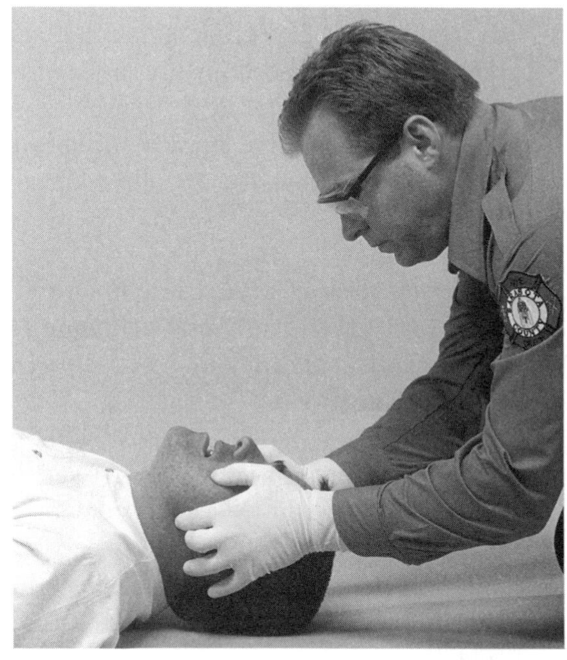

Figure 2-2c One-person bag valve mask

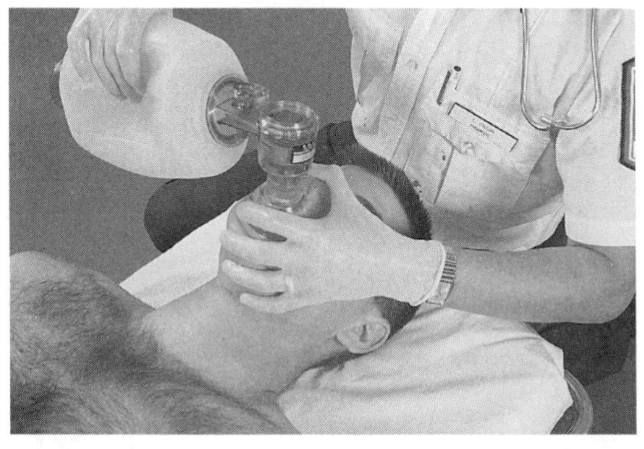

Figure 2-2d Two-person bag valve mask technique

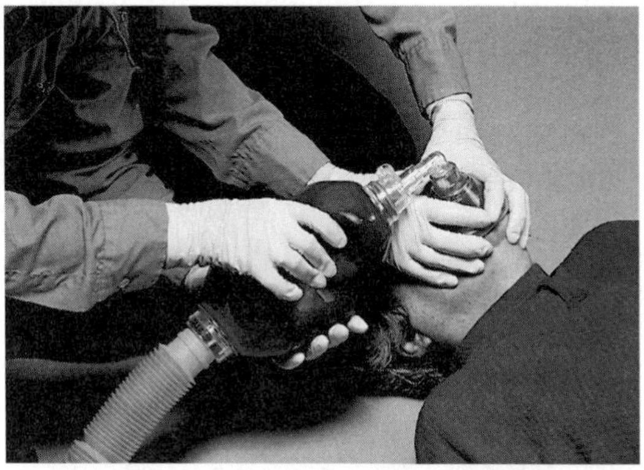

Figure 2-2e Cricoid pressure

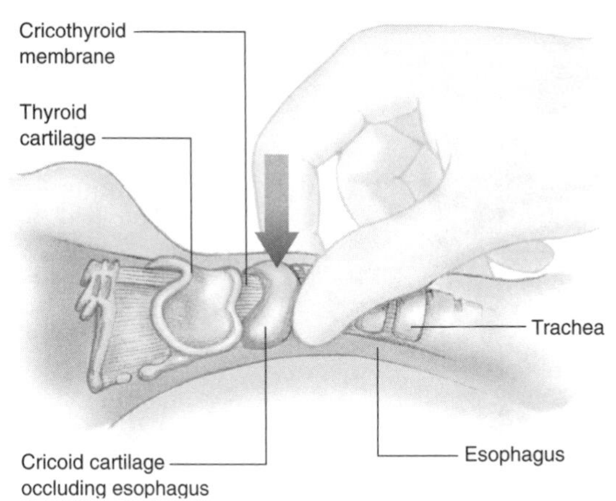

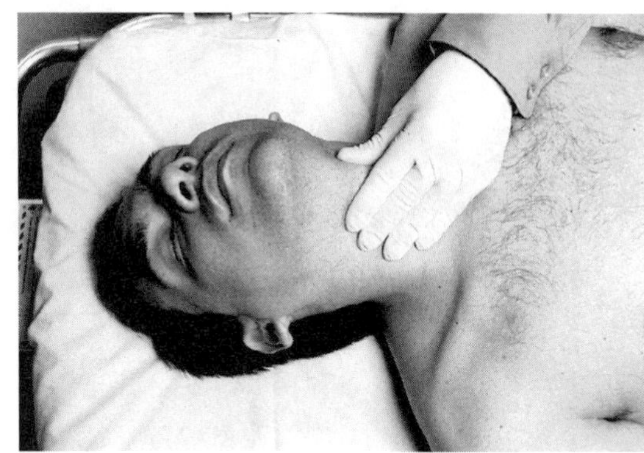

advanced skills. If a clinician skilled and competent in advanced airway procedures is not readily available it is preferable to continue bag valve mask ventilations rather than attempt to use other airway devices.

Maintaining the Airway While Using the Bag Valve Mask or for Patients Whose Mentation Is Diminished to the Point They Do Not Maintain Their Own Airway

1. Oral Pharyngeal Airway (OPA). Used in patients with no gag reflex. This device is inserted behind the tongue to keep the tongue from falling back into the posterior pharynx and causing the epiglottis to occlude the airway.

   Insertion is accomplished by moving the tongue forward with a tongue blade and sliding the device anatomically behind the tongue (Figure 2-3). Alternatively the device can be placed back into the airway as far as possible at a 90° or 180° angle, then rotated to rest behind the tongue. OPAs come in various sizes. The proper size is assured by measuring against the patient's exterior anatomy. The appropriate size reaches from the angle of the jaw to the corner. This is only used in unconscious patients who have no gag reflex.
2. Nasal Pharyngeal Airways (NPA). Used in patients who require airway assistance but still have an intact gag reflex or the inability to open their mouth. This device also keeps the tongue from falling against the posterior pharynx and occluding the airway.

   Insertion: The device is sized similar to the oral airway. The NPA comes In various sizes; choose the one that extends from the angle of the jaw to the tip of the nose. The device is inserted (Figure 2-4) by lubricating it liberally, then inserting the NPA into the nare in a posterior fashion (towards the back of the throat).

   The NPA is flexible and will bend to follow the nasal pharynx to lodge behind the tongue. The beveled edge is designed to be placed towards the septum. The NPA is designed for the right nare if it is to be placed in using the anatomical position.

   If the left nare is used, the NPA must be placed in backwards (facing upwards),

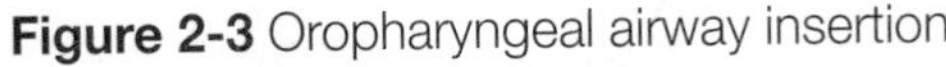
Figure 2-3 Oropharyngeal airway insertion

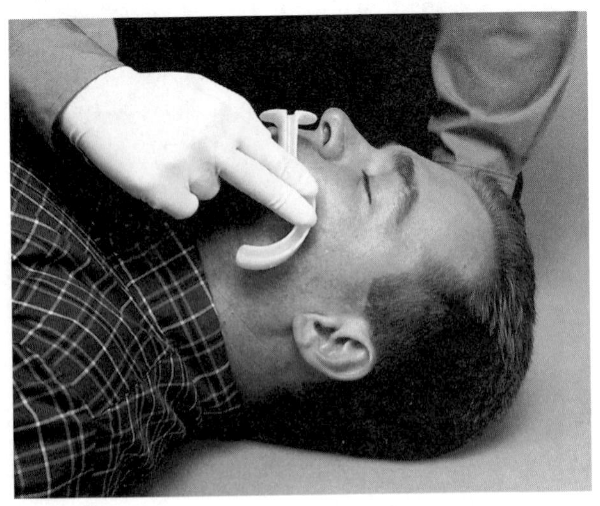

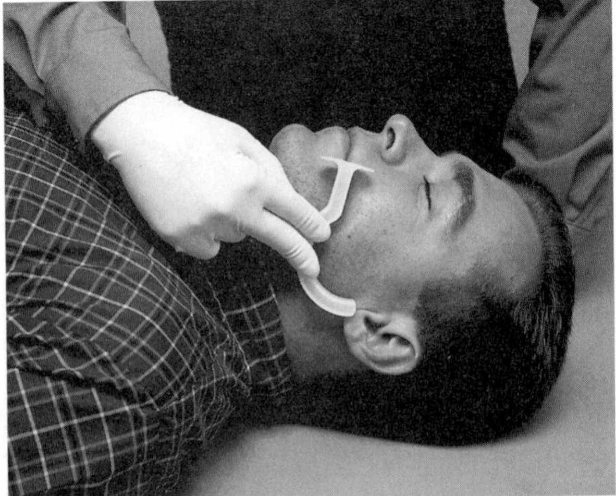

Figure 2-3 *(Continued)*

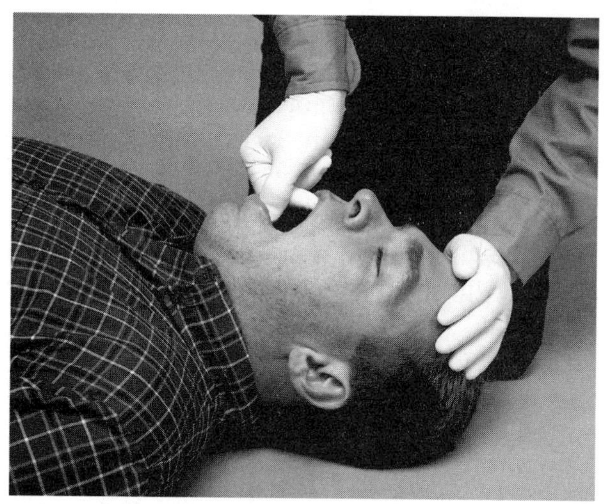

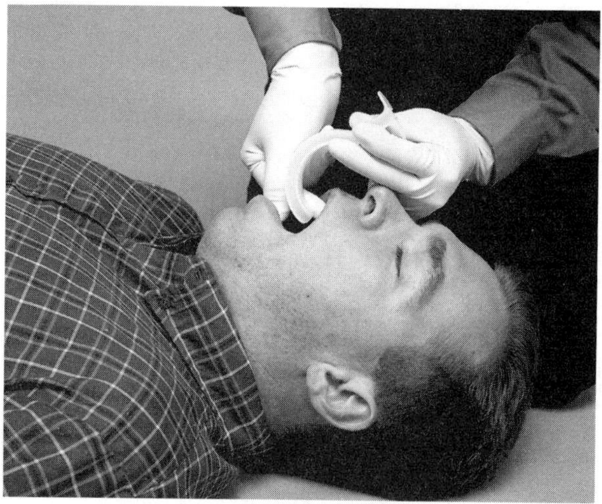

Figure 2-4 Nasopharyngeal airway insertion

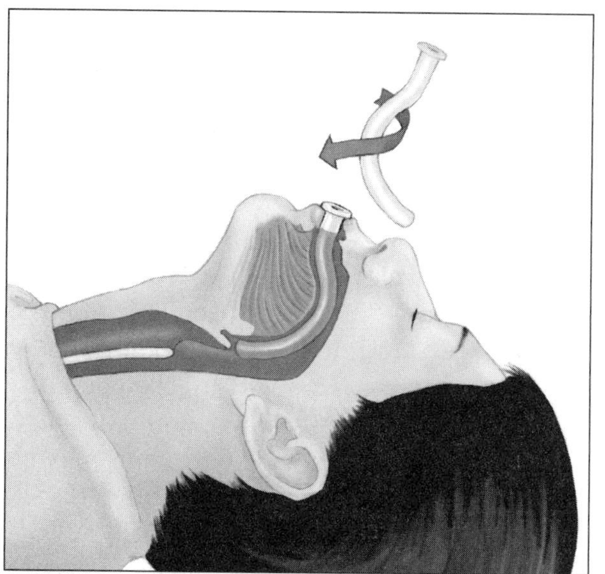

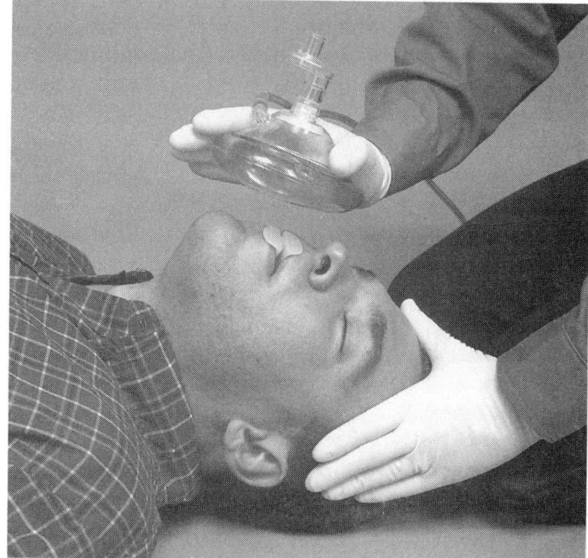

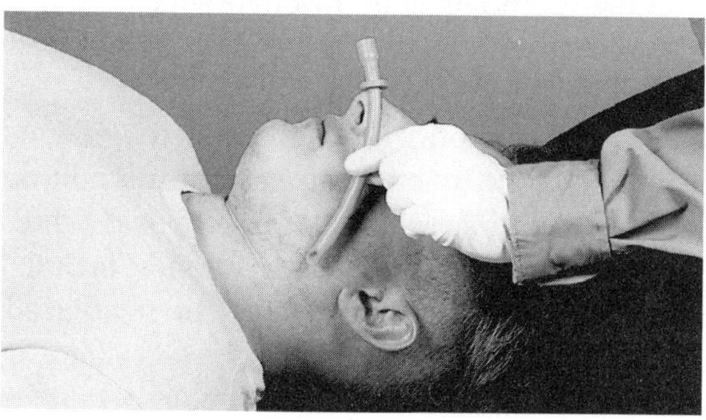

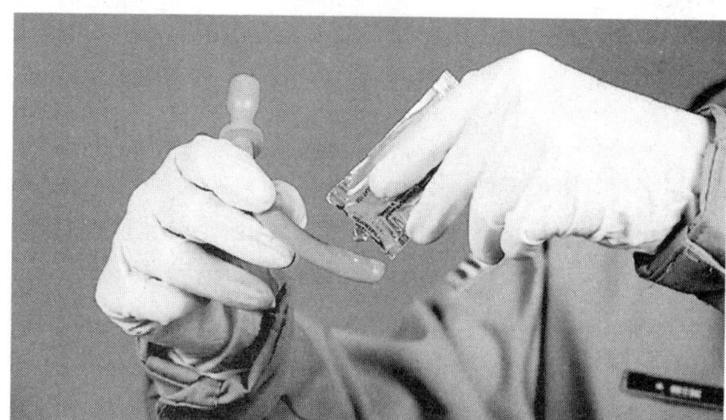

Figure 2-4 *(Continued)*

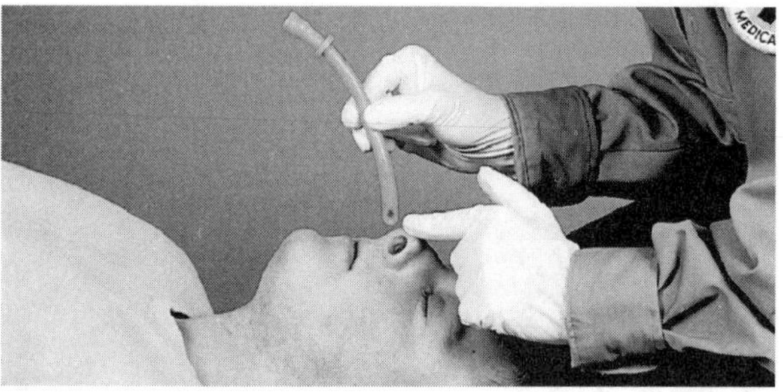

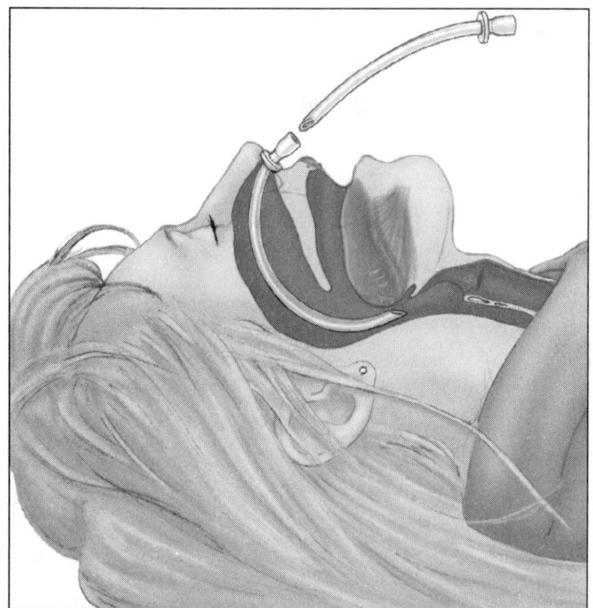

then rotated as it reaches the posterior pharynx. *Warning:* Do not use NPAs on patients who display signs of a basilar skull fracture (blood or CSF from the ears or nose following head trauma) as there is a slight potential it could enter the cranial vault.

ENDOTRACHEAL INTUBATION

Placing a cuffed tube into the trachea is the preferred method of airway control only for those who are **skilled** at the procedure; intubation should not cause a delay in providing CPR and other ACLS procedures. Intubation is indicated in patients who suffer respiratory or cardiac arrest or who are unconscious to the point they are not able to protect their airway with a gag reflex. Tracheal intubation provides a secured airway, reduces the potential for aspiration, allows for oxygen delivery at 100%, and may provide an optional, though minimally effective, drug route if need be (NAVEL: Narcan, Atropine, Vasopressin, Epinephrine, and Lidocaine can be given via the ET tube at 2–2½ times the IV dose, but should only be given if there is no IV or intraosseous access). Intubation should be attempted only in patients who have been initially ventilated by other means. Intubation should only be done by those qualified and skilled in the procedure. Bag valve mask ventilation or other less invasive airway devices (discussed later) are effective and acceptable as long as the provider is competent in their use and the device is supplying adequate emergency ventilation as evidenced by chest rise with each ventilation.

INTUBATION EQUIPMENT

1. Laryngoscope handle and appropriate type and size blade. The curved blade (Macintosh #3 or #4 for adults) is used to put pressure into the valecula at the base of the tongue. This will lift the epiglottis to expose the glottic opening through which the trachea and vocal cords may be viewed. The straight blade (Miller #2, #3, or #4 for adults) is used to directly visualize and gently lift the epiglottis to expose the glottic opening through which the trachea and vocal cords may be viewed (Figure 2-5).
2. Cuffed endotracheal tube. Sized by diameter in millimeters. In general, for adults, 7.0–8.0 mm is used for females, while 7.5–8.5 mm is appropriate for most males.
3. Stylette. A stiffener that can be placed inside the ET tube to give the tube shape if needed.

Figure 2-5a The curved blade lifts the vallecula

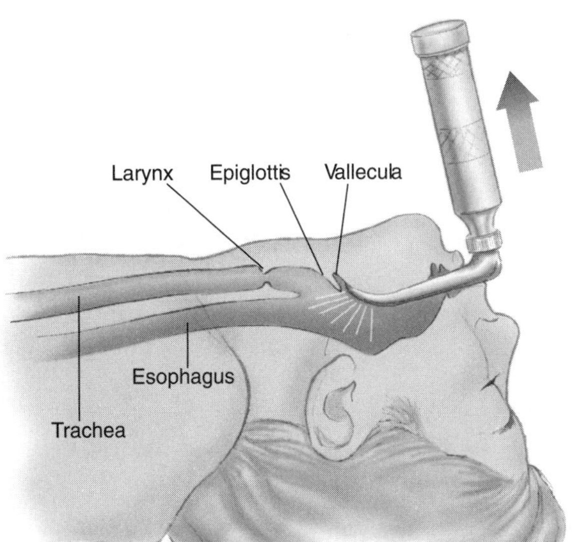

Figure 2-5b The straight blade lifts the epiglottis

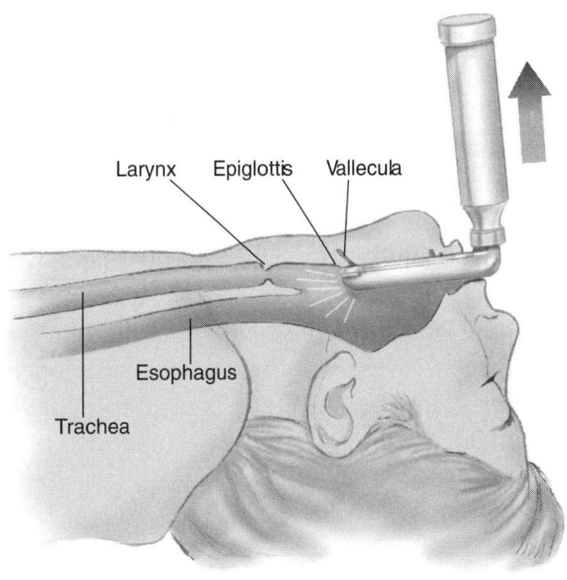

Figure 2-5c (A) Stylet and (B) stylet in place

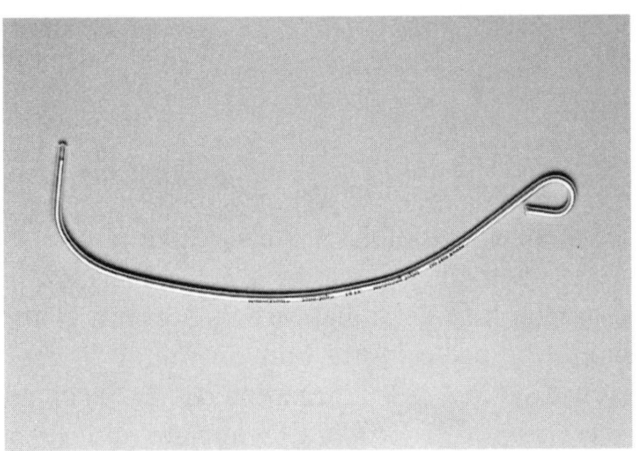

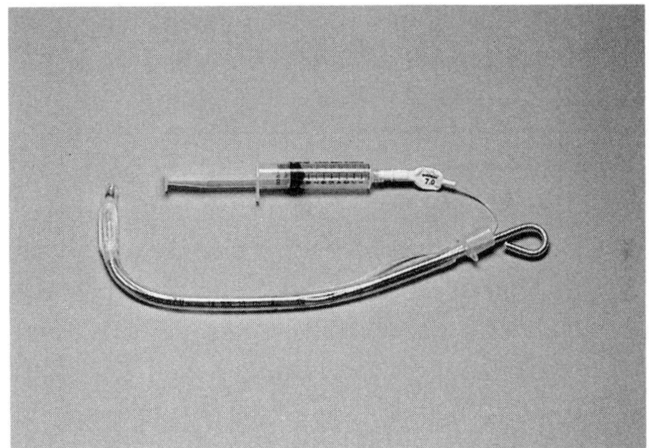

4. Syringe to inflate the ET tube cuff with 5–10 cc of air.
5. Tube confirmation and securing devices (discussed later).

Intubation procedure: Have suction ready to clear the airway of any secretions. Intubation should not exceed 30 seconds without ventilations and should only be attempted by those who are authorized, skilled, and proficient in advanced airway procedures. Gentle cricoid pressure similar to that recommended during bag valve mask ventilation may increase the intubator's view by moving the larynx posteriorly for better alignment with the oral pharynx.

1. Position the patient properly. Begin with the standard sniffing position to open the airway as you ventilate with the bag valve mask. Patients are unique—some tracheas are better viewed by hyperextending the neck, some by elevating the occiput, and some fall

somewhere between the two. The patient's unique anatomy and the intubator's experience, technique, and skill will dictate exactly which position works best.

2. With the laryngoscope in the left hand, the intubator positions at the head and gently begins sliding the blade down the throat along the tongue. At the base of the tongue is the epiglottis. The curved blade will slide into the valecula (the space at the base of the tongue) and when the blade is lifted forward will expose the glottic opening. The straight blade is used to actually place under the epiglottis and lift it to expose the trachea.

Quick Tip

The laryngoscope is used to lift the tongue upward, not rock back on the teeth as this will break the teeth. Intubation takes much more training and skill than can be accomplished during an ACLS course.

3. The tracheal tube should have been prepared by placing the stylette into the tube (do not let the end of the wire stylette protrude past the end of the tracheal tube as this may cause soft tissue damage) and testing the cuff for leaks by inflating with 5 cc of air. The tube should be kept sterile. Once the laryngoscope is used to visualize the glottic opening and vocal cords the tube is passed from the right corner of the mouth, using the right hand, into the trachea. It is important to watch the tube enter the trachea. Insert the tube until the cuff is approximately one-half an inch past the vocal cords, which are visualized just past the glottic opening. The tube is generally placed to a depth of 21–25 cm at the lips as marked on the side of the ET tube. This depth generally keeps the tube past the vocal cords but above the carina and right main stem bronchus.

Figure 2-6 Glottic opening and vocal chords

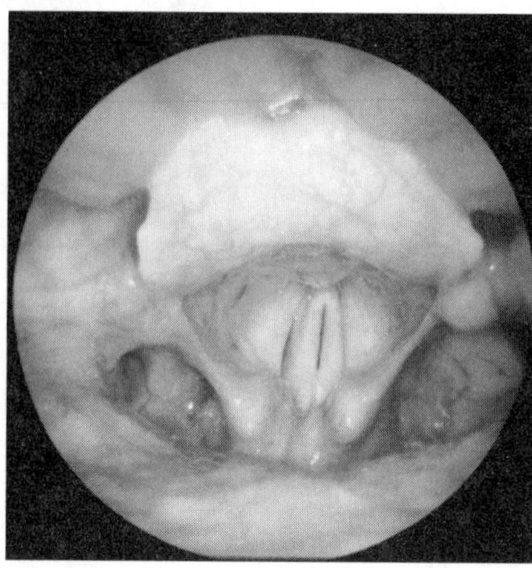

Remove the laryngoscope with the left hand and continually hold onto the tracheal tube until the tube is evaluated and secured. Inflate the cuff with 5–10 cc of air, then carefully remove the stylette, apply the bag valve mask, and begin ventilating the patient while evaluating for tube placement (Figure 2-6).

EVALUATING TRACHEAL TUBE POSITION

No method is foolproof. An ET tube left in an area other than the trachea (esophagus or hypopharynx) is a catastrophic event. Care should be taken to use both an initial clinical evaluation *and* a "confirmation device" such as an esophageal detector or CO_2 monitor (discussed later). ET tube placement should be continually evaluated throughout the resuscitation and postresuscitation phase of patient management. Anytime tube placement is in question, the patient should be extubated and reventilated before another intubation attempt with a fresh ET tube is started.

1. Listen over the epigastrium as you begin to ventilate the patient. Air heard in the stomach generally indicates the ET tube has been placed into the esophagus or hypopharyngeal area and should be removed.

2. Watch for chest rise and listen for air in the mid axillary and anterior lung fields as the patient is being ventilated. Both sides should sound roughly the same. More prominent breath sounds on the right generally indicates the tube was placed too deeply and is in the right main stem bronchus. In this case the tube should be gently pulled back until bilateral lung sounds are obtained. Monitor the depth of the ET tube and continually maintain its position. The goal is to keep the tube at a level that provides equal breath sounds and air movement as each side of the chest is auscultated.
3. Condensation seen in the tracheal tube as the patient exhales may be a clue the tube is in the trachea but, again, is not 100% reliable.
4. The most important and most reliable clinical evaluation comes when the provider who performed the intubation actually visualizes the ET tube in the trachea.

CONFIRMATION DEVICES

Along with evaluating clinical signs, assurance utilizing a "confirmation device" should be accomplished to further validate ET tube placement as well as to continually monitor tube position. Keep in mind *none* of these devices is 100% accurate 100% of the time.

1. Exhaled CO_2 detectors. Devices placed on the end of the tracheal tube, between the ET tube and the bag valve mask. They rely on perfusion to the lungs to create CO_2, which can be detected by color change, numeric value, or waveform depending on the complexity of the device. CO_2 detector devices are quite reliable in perfusing patients but may not give an adequate reading in the cardiac arrest victim due to minimal blood flow and poor CO_2 exchange at the lungs. The CO_2 detector should not be considered as a true "reading" until after 6 breaths have been given as residual CO_2 could be initially present in the esophagus.
2. Esophageal detector devices (EDD) are used to draw a negative pressure through the ET tube with a bulb or syringe type device. These devices are quite accurate (though not 100%) when used after the tracheal tube is placed, but before ventilations are given. These devices rely on the anatomy to help determine tube placement. The trachea is solid and supported by cartilage, thus suction applied to an ET tube that has been placed in the trachea will cause the detector device to fill with air. On the other hand, the device will not draw air if the tube is in the esophagus, as the esophagus is collapsible and will fold around the distal end of the tracheal tube and not allow air to pass. This EDD is the preferred initial device to help evaluate tube placement in the patient suffering cardiac arrest as it does not require perfusion (as opposed to CO_2 monitors) for accuracy (Figure 2-7).

Figure 2-7a Esophageal detector device

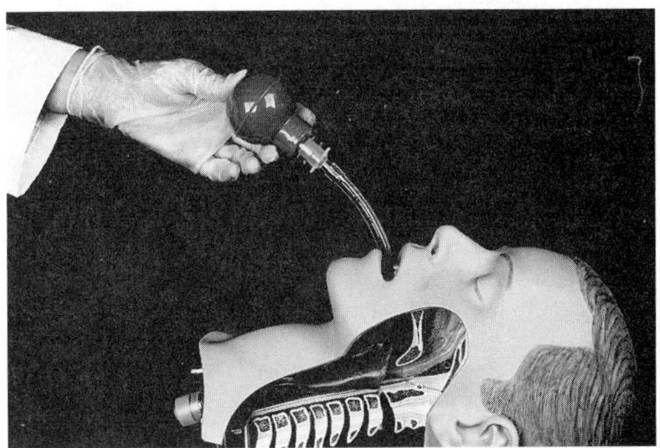

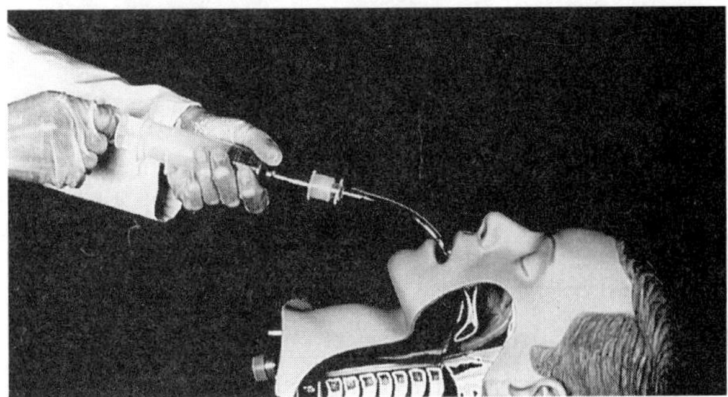

Figure 2-7b Electronic CO_2 capnometry

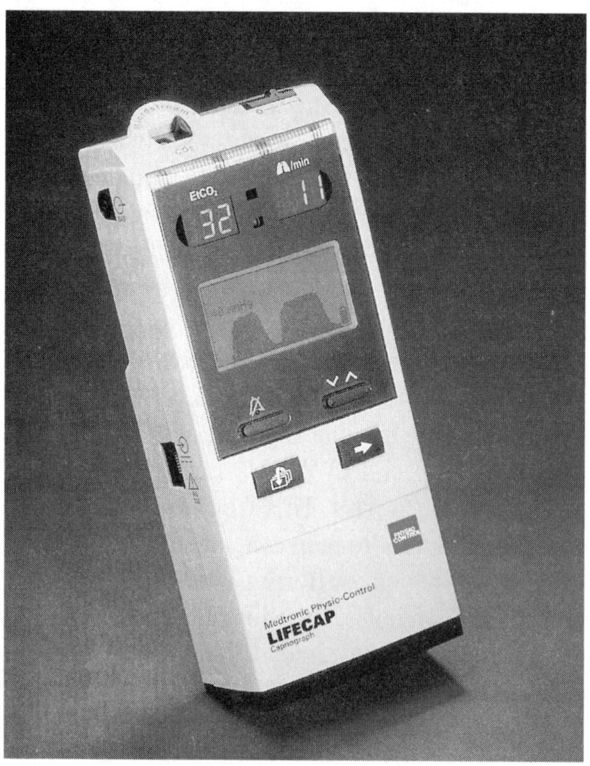

Figure 2-7c Colormetric CO_2 detector

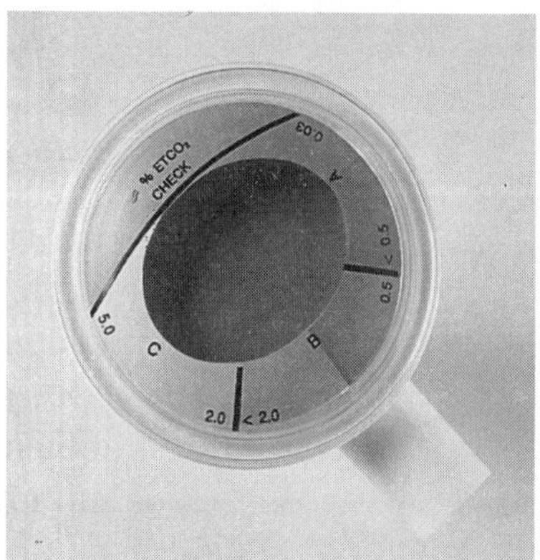

SECURING THE TRACHEAL TUBE

A commercial tracheal tube holder with built-in bite block is recommended; however, taping the tube and placing an oral airway back into the patient's mouth may also suffice. It may be prudent to immobilize the patient's head to reduce the possibility of tube dislodgement during transport or patient movement.

ALTERNATIVE AIRWAY DEVICES

These devices provide an alternative to the sometimes difficult skill of intubation for providers who are trained in and authorized to use them. These devices may be indicated for patients in whom intubation has been unsuccessful, or used as the primary method of airway control following bag valve mask ventilations by rescuers who are not able to be trained or not able to keep up intubation skills. Again, these devices are not foolproof and before use require training, skill, and authorization depending on your professional license.

1. Esophageal tracheal Combitube™. Designed for adults only, this device is blindly inserted past the posterior pharynx and generally seats in the esophagus (Figure 2-8a). The tube actually has two ventilation ports and will function whether the tube was placed in

Figure 2-8a Esophageal tracheal Combitube

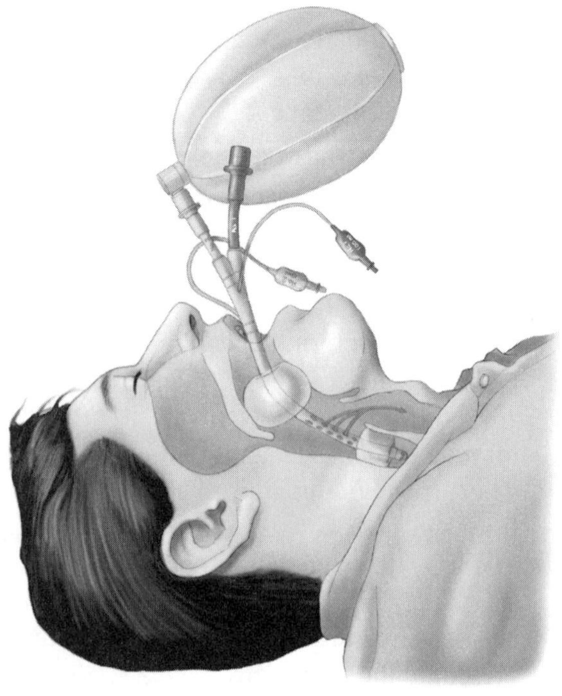

Figure 2-8b Laryngeal mask airway (LMA)

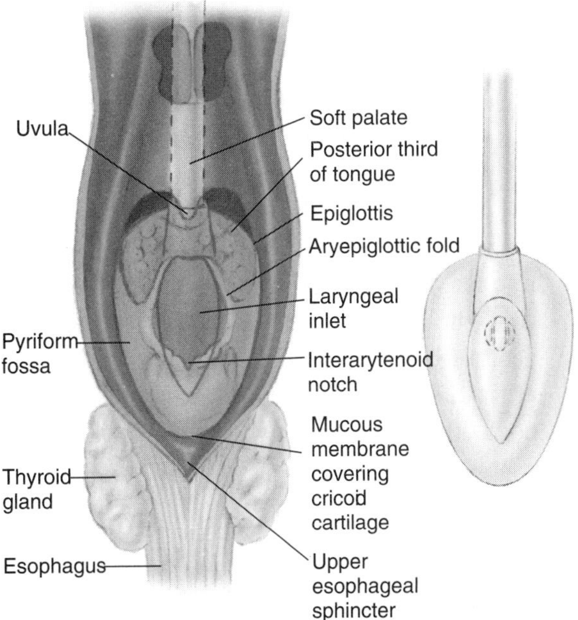

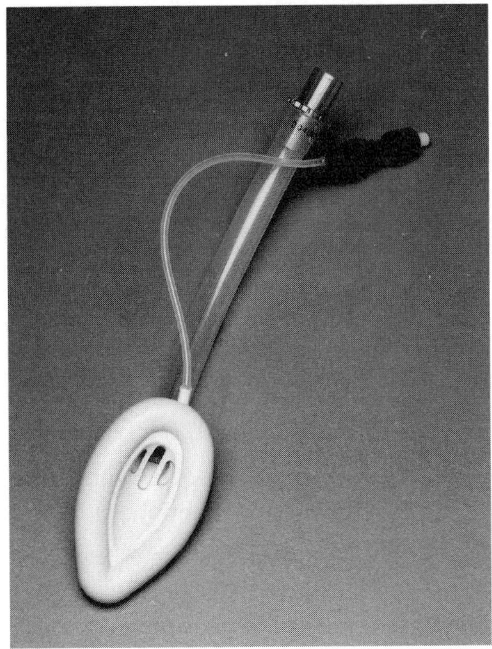

the esophagus or inadvertently placed in the trachea by simply ventilating through whichever tube causes chest rise and lung sounds without gastric inflation. The Combitube is used only in adults with no gag reflex who require ventilatory support. The device is contraindicated in patients under 5′ tall or 16 years old, or patients who are prone to have significant bleeding from the esophagus such as esophageal disease or caustic ingestion.

2. Laryngeal mask airway (LMA). This device consists of a tube with a cuffed masklike end, which is blindly inserted into the pharynx by gently sliding it down the back of the throat while following the curvature and holding the device against the roof of the mouth and posterior pharynx as it is pushed into place (Figure 2-8b). As the device is introduced in the pharynx, its shape will cause it to "stop" as it reaches the area of the glottic opening. The cuff is then inflated, which causes the mask to seal against the glottic opening. This device is quick and fairly simple and protects the airway better than a bag valve mask alone. The device is sized from infant through adult based on weight. Like the Combitube, the LMA is indicated in patients with no gag reflex who require ventilatory support. The laryngeal mask airway cannot be used in patients with an intact gag reflex and should be used with caution in patients with active airway secretions or bleeding or vomiting as the device does not fully protect from aspiration. There are other variations of laryngeal airways produced by several manufacturers.

Quick Tip

Once any of the ventilation tube devices are placed, the respiration rate should be decreased to 8–10 breaths/min (about 1 breath every 6 seconds).

Practice Test—Airway Management

1. A patient in congestive heart failure with significant respiratory distress and a

respiratory rate of 28 should *initially* receive oxygen by what means:

A. Nasal cannula.
B. Nonrebreather face mask.
C. Immediate intubation.
D. An oral pharyngeal airway.

2. In relation to providing ventilation to a nonbreathing adult:

A. Intubation should be the initial priority for every ACLS provider.
B. Providing the head tilt–chin lift will not open the airway.
C. It is preferred to continue slow bag valve mask ventilations until a skilled intubator arrives.
D. A bag valve mask should not be used in patients with bradycardia.

3. Providing cricoid pressure during ventilations will:

A. Keep the heart rate regular.
B. Reduce the chance of an oxygen ventilation mismatch.
C. Keep the patient from moving too much.
D. Reduce gastric filling and vomiting potential.

4. You are resuscitating a 62-year-old female who collapsed in the mall. She has been successfully intubated. The rate at which she should be ventilated is:

A. Whatever rate maintains an oxygen saturation of 96%.
B. 30–32 breaths per minute.
C. 8–10 breaths per minute.
D. 3–4 breaths per kilogram of body weight.

5. The appropriate sequence for providing ventilations in the unconscious respiratory arrested patient is:

A. Position the head, apply the bag valve mask, ventilate slowly.
B. Hyperventilate, place a nasal airway, call for cricoid pressure.
C. Attempt nasal cannula, flex the head, bag valve mask slowly.
D. Immediate placement of an endotracheal tube, bag valve mask at 16 breaths per minute.

6. Once the skilled intubator has placed the tracheal tube through the glottic opening (into the trachea) the placement must be assessed. Which of the following is a clinical sign the tracheal tube has been correctly placed?

A. Air is heard over the epigastric region.
B. The chest rises each time the bag valve mask is squeezed.
C. The stomach rises each time the bag valve mask is squeezed.
D. The patient begins to gag on the tracheal tube.

7. Once the clinical evaluation of tracheal tube placement has been conducted and it is thought the tube has been correctly placed, what procedures should be accomplished next?

A. Tape the tube, hyperventilate, and apply suction.
B. Apply the ventilator, monitor blood pressure, and secure the tube.
C. Use a confirmation device such as a CO_2 detector, and a commercial device to secure the tracheal tube.
D. Each procedure will vary according to the patient's ECG rhythm.

8. Though, in the past, tracheal intubation has been thought of as the "gold standard" in airway control, several devices may be used to provide adequate and successful ventilations in patients in

whom intubation has been unsuccessful or by clinicians who have been trained in their use rather than intubation. These devices may include:

A. Esophageal or laryngeal airways.
B. Triple lumen tubes.
C. Bag valve trachea laryngeal tubes.
D. Hypopharyngeal gastric tube airways.

9. An intubated patient must be carried on the stretcher down a flight of stairs. Which of the following should be accomplished in order to help maintain the ET tube in the proper position?
   A. Immobilize the patient's head and neck.
   B. Nothing needs to be done so long as the ET tube cuff is inflated.
   C. Push the ET tube 2 cm deeper into the trachea.
   D. Use a loop double tape technique.

10. You have received a patient who is lying in bed. The patient is slightly cyanotic and seems to take an occasional agonal breath but has no regular or effective breathing. You determine he is unresponsive and call for assistance. The first step to assure the patient has a patent airway should be to:
    A. Attempt to ventilate.
    B. Call for the Combitube or laryngeal mask airway.
    C. Place the patient into the sniffing position.
    D. Begin bag mask ventilations at 20 breaths per minute.

11. As you attempt to ventilate a 60-year-old overweight victim of sudden cardiac arrest, you realize you are having difficulty maintaining head position and obtaining adequate chest rise as the tongue continues to fall into the posterior pharynx. Which type of device may be useful in assisting to maintain this patient's airway?
    A. A glottic airway device.
    B. More aggressive bag valve mask ventilations.
    C. Slower bag valve mask ventilations.
    D. An oral pharyngeal airway (OPA).

12. A patient experiencing mild to moderate chest pain with mild respiratory distress and adequate oxygen saturation should receive oxygen initially by what means?
    A. Nonrebreather mask.
    B. Venturi mask.
    C. Nasal cannula.
    D. Oxygen is not necessary in this case.

13. You respond to a cardiac arrest victim. The entire team is with the patient and all equipment is available. In reference to attempting to intubate this patient, when is the appropriate time?
    A. Immediately as airway is the most important skill.
    B. After the second defibrillation.
    C. Once the IV is patent.
    D. Only after effective ventilations have been established with a bag valve mask.

14. Which is correct in relation to bag valve mask ventilation?
    A. Bag valve mask ventilation is effective and can provide nearly 100% oxygen.
    B. Bag valve mask ventilation is of little value and should be withheld for intubation.
    C. Bag valve mask ventilation is a skill reserved for EMTs only.
    D. The latest guidelines recommend intubation prior to bag valve mask.

15. In relation to the Combitube esophageal type and the laryngeal mask type airways, the ACLS guidelines state:
    A. These devices have no place in respiratory management, and should not be considered.
    B. These devices are effective and provide an option to intubation for those trained and authorized to use them.
    C. These devices should only be used after several minutes of intubation have failed.
    D. Providers should routinely consider this their initial means of ventilation control.

16. The physician has intubated a patient following an episode of ventricular fibrillation. The patient currently has a pulse and heart rate of 110 per minute and blood pressure of 98/50 but remains apneic. The provider who is evaluating the chest cannot positively identify lung sounds by auscultation of the chest though it appears the chest and epigastric region are rising each time the patient is ventilated. The CO_2 monitor is detecting a level of zero. The most prudent action to perform based on these findings is:
    A. Increase the rate and volume of ventilations with the bag valve mask.
    B. Put the patient on a ventilator.
    C. Extubate the patient and immediately ventilate with a bag valve mask.
    D. Apply a pulse oximeter to evaluate the patient's oxygen saturation.

17. During cardiac arrest, along with clinical evaluation, which device is most effective initially to help evaluate endotracheal tube placement?
    A. Esophageal detector device.
    B. CO_2 monitor.
    C. Esophageal Combitube airway.
    D. Oral pharyngeal airway.

18. Which of the following may an assistant do to help during a difficult intubation?
    A. Provide suction to clear the airway of secretions.
    B. Help properly position the head.
    C. Apply gently cricoid pressure.
    D. All of the above.

19. The respiratory therapist had been bag valve mask ventilating a 70-year-old stroke victim with respiratory depression for the past 5 minutes. The patient is not maintaining his own airway as evident by the fact he is not gagging on an appropriately placed oral pharyngeal airway; thus the physician requests the patient be intubated. What is the appropriate size ET tube to use for this patient?
    A. Tube size will be based on the patient's weight.
    B. 7.5–8.5mm endotracheal tube.
    C. 21–25 cm tube.
    D. 10–12mm endotracheal tube.

20. A patient was intubated by paramedics and flown to your facility. Their medical chart documents the ET tube was originally placed at 23 cm depth at the patient's lip. Currently you note the tube to be at 28 cm at the lip. The most common complication of change in tube depth is:
    A. The endotracheal tube was pulled from the trachea.
    B. The endotracheal tube was pushed into the right mainstem bronchus.
    C. The tracheal tube has perforated the esophagus.
    D. This few centimeters is not a significant finding.

CHAPTER

3 ECG Review

Cardiac Monitoring

Continuous cardiac monitoring allows us to watch someone's electrical cardiac activity over a period of time. Monitoring may be used, among other things, to:

- Look for causes for clinical signs and symptoms—for example, syncopal episodes, palpitations, hypotension.
- Monitor the frequency of cardiac arrhythmias and be able to treat them in a timely manner.
- Monitor the effectiveness of medications.

Cardiac monitoring tells us about the electrical activity of the heart. Electrical information is transmitted through the skin via electrodes to a monitor, which translates the electrical impulses into waveforms that we can see and can be drawn on paper. On the ECG screen we see a representation of the electrical activity of the heart. It's not until we assess the patient that we get information regarding the mechanical activity of the heart.

Cardiac monitoring is definitely a "garbage in–garbage out" situation. If the monitor doesn't receive good information through the skin via the electrodes, then the picture on the screen and the decisions that can be made based on that are less than optimal.

Two major factors in the quality of your ECG tracing are *electrode placement,* and *quality of skin/electrode contact.*

ELECTRODE PLACEMENT

For continuous monitoring, there are 3-, 4-, and 5-lead systems. Originally, when monitoring heart patients, leads were placed on the extremities and the chest; now, although placement is modified, the abbreviations remain: RA (right arm), LA (left arm), LL (left leg), RL (right leg), C (chest).

These electrodes are usually color-coded:

RA	white
LA	black
LL	red
RL	green
C	brown

If three electrodes are used, placement looks like Figure 3-1.

Quick Tip

Remember: White on the right, black opposite white, red on the ribs.

Contact Between Skin and Electrodes

To get good conduction of impulses through the electrodes, there should be maximum contact between the skin and electrodes. Ideally, the electrodes should remain packaged until use, so the conductive gel remains moist. Dry, cracked gel doesn't conduct well.

The skin should be prepared to encourage a good "stick":

- Dry skin that is wet or diaphoretic.

Figure 3-1 ECG electrode placement

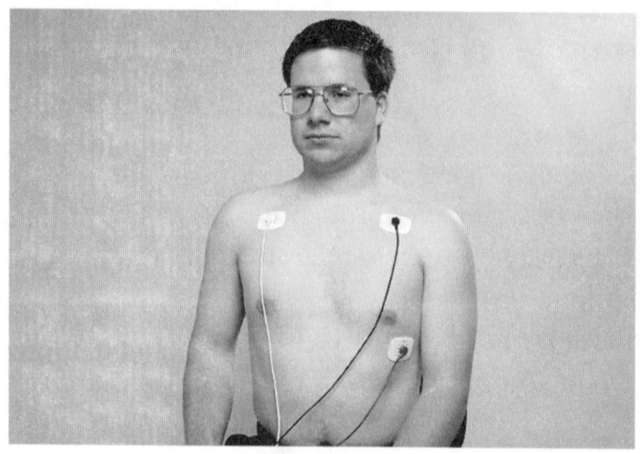

- Wash and dry skin that is oily.
- Remove hair at electrode site.
- Do not place electrodes over medication patches or implanted devices.
- Slightly abrade the skin with a washcloth or, if available, the bumpy underside of the electrode backing.
- Avoid tension on the electrode wires.

Other factors:

- Movement can interfere with the electrode signal:
  - If the red electrode is placed on a part of the chest that moves with respiration, your ECG tracing may have a wavy baseline.
  - If your patient is shivering, seizing, ambulating, wiggling his ECG cables, or moving around in bed, you may see artifact on the screen that makes it difficult to analyze the rhythm.

Analyzing Rhythms

When naming rhythms, we typically answer two questions:

- Where in the heart does this rhythm originate?
- How is the heart rate?

To come to these conclusions, ask the following questions about each rhythm that you look at:

- Is it regular?
  - Are the R-R intervals all the same?
  - If the R-R is not regular, is there one beat causing the irregularity, or is the irregularity throughout the strip?
- What is the rate?
  - Consider the atrial (P-wave) as well as the ventricular (QRS complex) rate.
- How are the Ps?
  - Can you find them?
  - Are they upright?
  - Do they all look the same?
  - Is each P wave followed by a QRS complex?
  - Does each QRS complex have a P-wave?

- What is the PR interval?
- How wide is the QRS complex?
- Are there any out-of-the-ordinary beats that should be described after you name the underlying rhythm?
  - Where in the heart do they originate?
  - How are they timed? Are they early beats or late beats?

When looking at rhythms, we compare what we see to what is normal:

NORMAL SINUS RHYTHM

Sinus (SA) node is the pacemaker creating upright P-waves (Figure 3-2).

REGULARITY:	The rhythm is regular.
RATE:	The atrial and ventricular rates are equal: 60–100. Rate <60—sinus bradycardia; rate >100—sinus tachycardia.

Figure 3-2 Normal sinus rhythm (NSR)

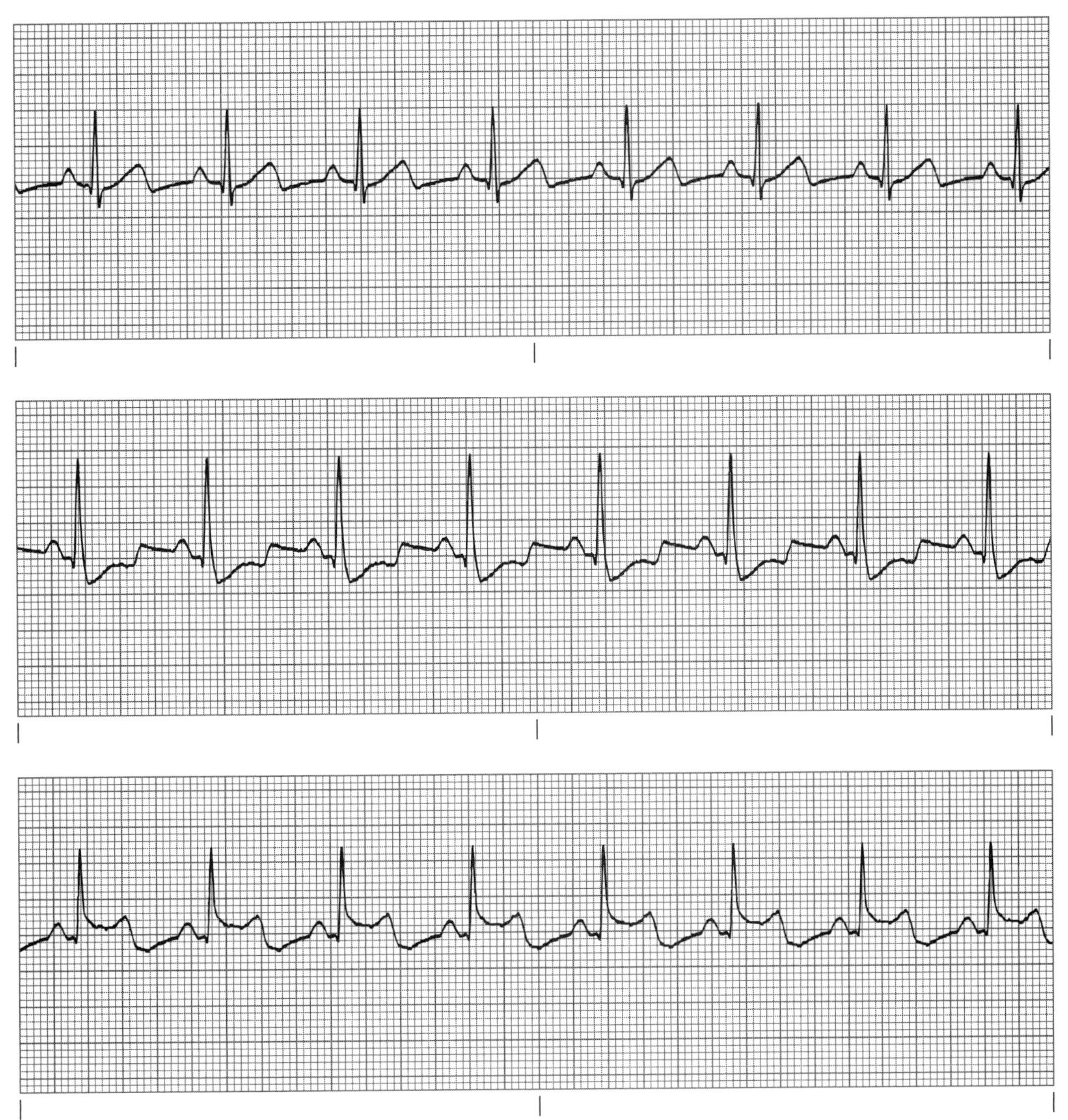

P-WAVES:	The P-waves are uniform. There is one P for each QRS.
PRI:	0.12 to 0.20 seconds—constant.
QRS:	Less than 0.12 seconds.

BRADYCARDIAS

Bradycardia means "slow heart." A slow heart rate is a problem for the patient if the rate is not fast enough to adequately deliver oxygenated blood to important organ systems, so bradycardias are treated if the patient is symptomatic. There are many parameters that can be assessed to help determine if the patient is symptomatic. Objective parameters include mental status, blood pressure, chest pain, and lung sounds. If there are significant changes in any of these findings, then the patient may be considered symptomatic. More subjective (but also helpful!) findings might include pallor, weakness, diaphoresis, or cool extremities.

Your patient may have an absolute bradycardia, where his heart rate is less than 60 beats per minute, or a relative bradycardia, where the heart rate is too slow for the clinical picture. The most important factor is the patient's response to the heart rate.

Exact rhythm diagnosis is helpful, but remember, "Treat the patient, not the monitor." The most important questions to ask about a patient with a rhythm that may cause a bradycardia are:

Is the patient's heart rate slow?

Is the patient symptomatic?

Rhythms that may be bradycardic:

Sinus Bradycardia

The sinus (SA) node is the pacemaker creating upright P-waves (Figure 3-3).

Figure 3-3 Sinus bradycardia (SB)

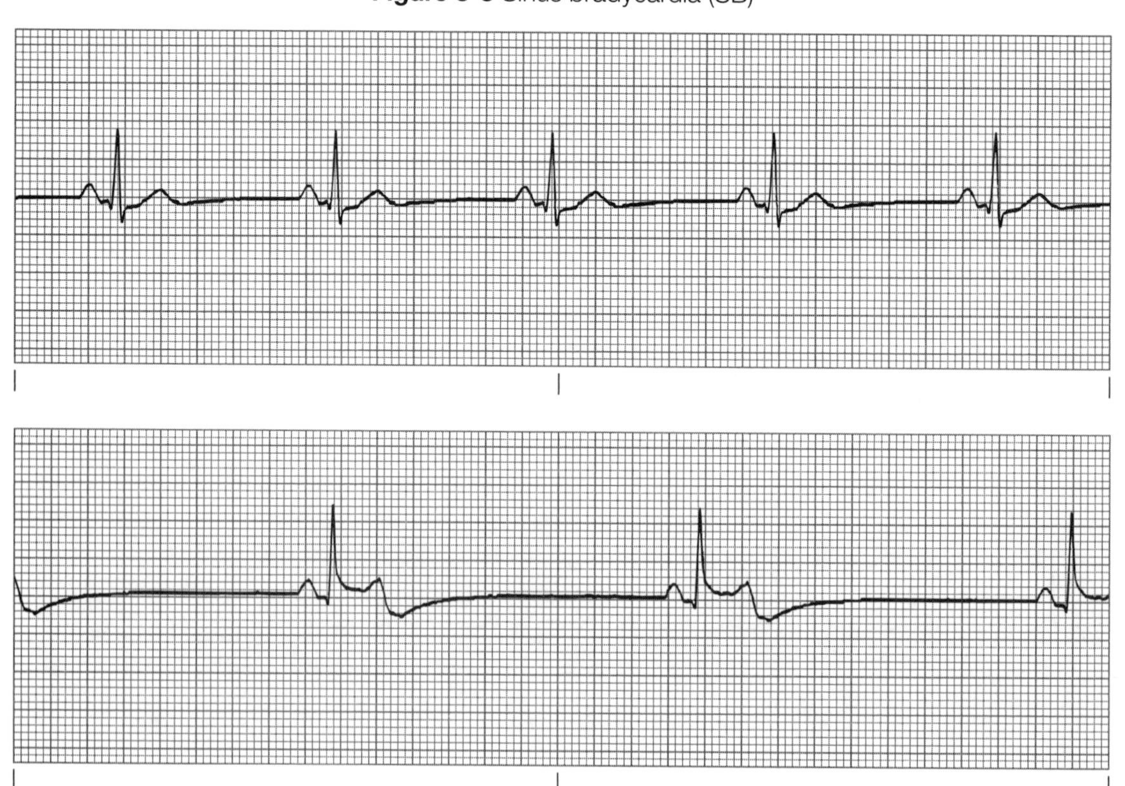

REGULARITY: The rhythm is regular.
RATE: The atrial and ventricular rates are equal and less than 60 per minute.
P-WAVES: The P-waves are uniform. There is one P for each QRS.
PRI: 0.12 to 0.20 seconds—constant.
QRS: Less than 0.12 seconds.

Junctional Escape Rhythm

When higher pacemaker sites fail, the AV junction takes over (Figure 3-4). The atria are depolarized via retrograde (backwards or "uphill") conduction. Ventricular conduction is normal.

REGULARITY: The rhythm is regular.
RATE: Usually 40–60
P-WAVES: If visible before the QRS complex, the P-wave will be inverted. If not visible, then the P-wave is hidden within the QRS complex, indicating that the atria and ventricles depolarize at the same time. An inverted P-wave may also be found following the QRS complex, indicating that the atria depolarize after the ventricles.
PRI: If the P-wave precedes the QRS complex, the

Figure 3-4 Junctional rhythm (JR)

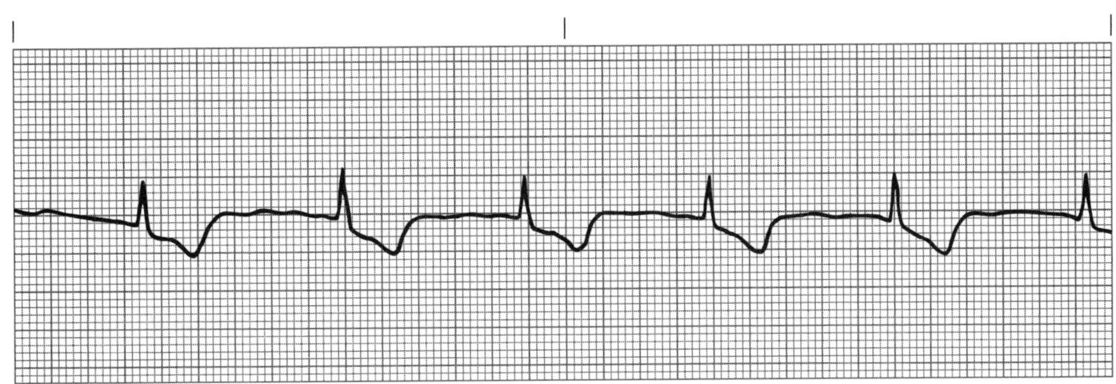

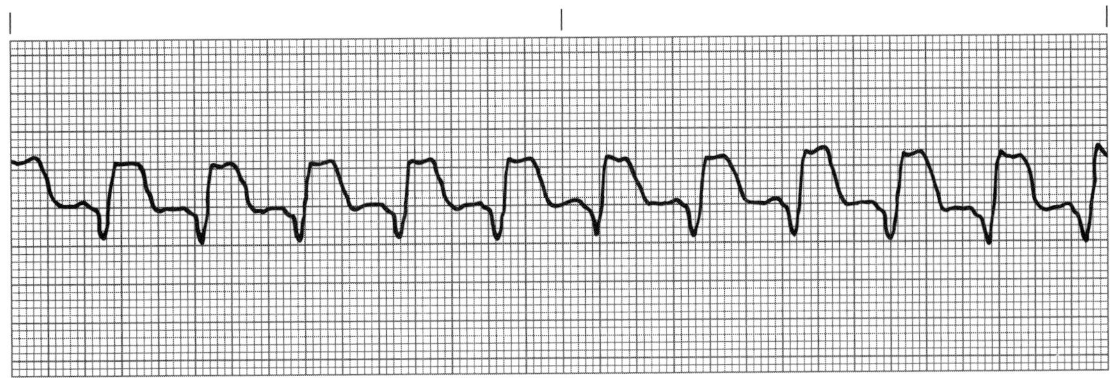

Figure 3-5 Idioventricular rhythm (IVR)

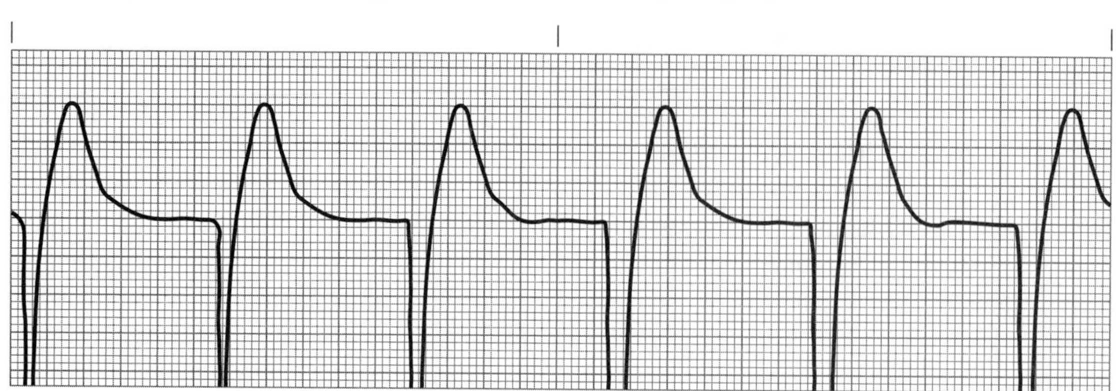

	PRI will be less than 0.20 seconds.
QRS:	Usually normal

Idioventricular Rhythm

In the absence of a higher pacemaker, the ventricles initiate a regular impulse at their inherent rate of 20–40 beats per minute (Figure 3-5).

REGULARITY:	Rhythm is regular.
RATE:	Usually 20–40 beats per minute (rate between 40 and 100 beats per minute would be called accelerated idioventricular rhythm).
P-WAVES:	No P-waves.
PRI:	Not measurable since there is no P-wave.
QRS:	The QRS complex is wide and bizarre.

Quick Tip

Remember: "The lower you go, the slower it goes." Pacemakers low in the heart generally have lower intrinsic rates (AV junction: 40–60, Ventricles: 20–40).

Heart Blocks

Heart blocks are a concern in ACLS when impulses originating in the SA node are not properly conducted to the ventricles, causing a slow heart rate, and signs and symptoms of poor oxygen delivery (symptomatic bradycardia). Although the primary concern is whether the patient's heart rate is slow and he is symptomatic, a more definitive diagnosis of the block can help you choose the most effective therapy. There are four types of heart blocks:

First-Degree AV Block. In first-degree block, conduction through the AV node is slower than normal. Each impulse is eventually conducted, and once the impulse reaches the ventricles, conduction proceeds normally (Figure 3-6).

REGULARITY:	The rhythm is regular.
RATE:	The rate may vary, and the name of the underlying rhythm (sinus bradycardia, sinus tachycardia, sinus rhythm) is included before mentioning the first-degree block.
P-WAVES:	The P-waves are upright and uniform. Each P-wave is followed by a QRS complex.

Figure 3-6 First-Degree AV Block (1° AVB)

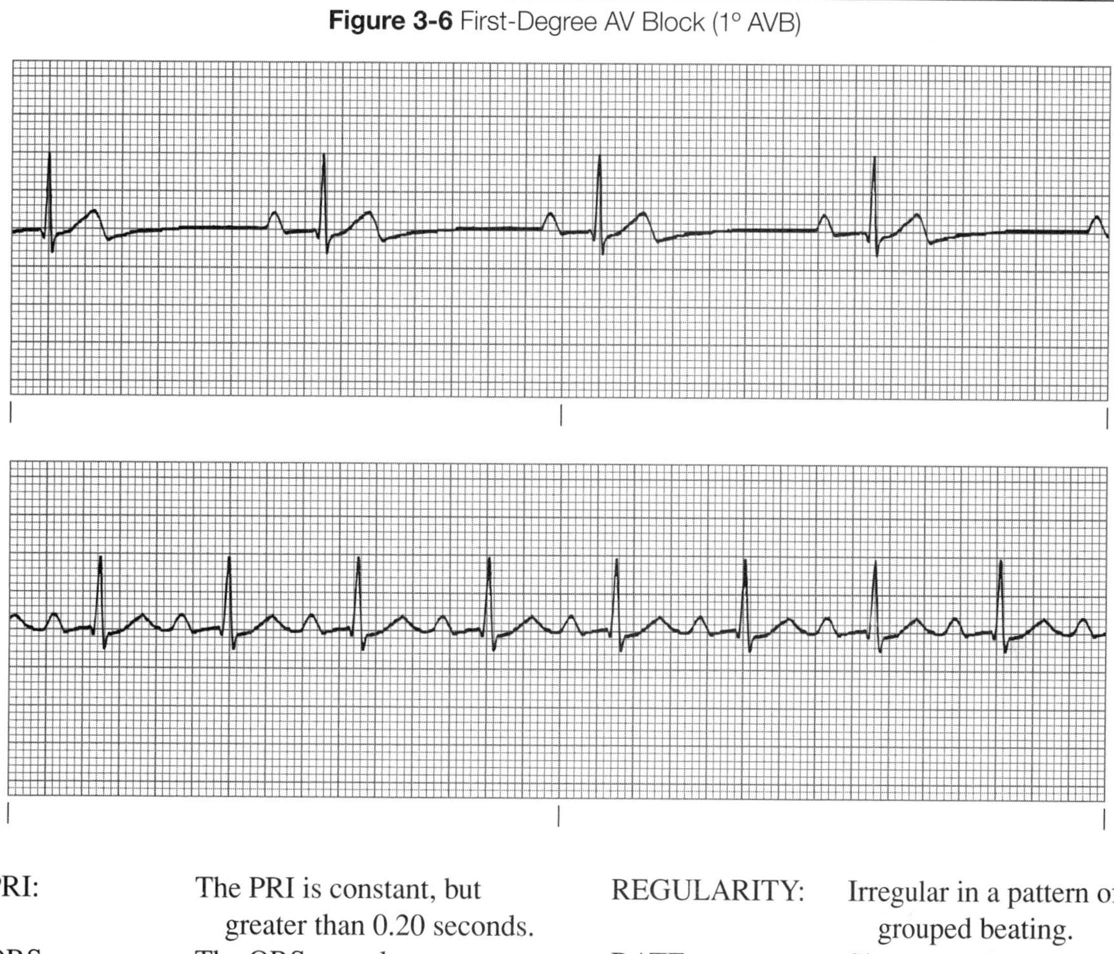

PRI: The PRI is constant, but greater than 0.20 seconds.

QRS: The QRS complex measurement is normal; less than 0.12 seconds

Second-Degree Heart Blocks. In second-degree heart blocks, not every impulse causing a P-wave is conducted down to the ventricles. This causes P-waves to appear on the monitor without a QRS complex. There are two types of second-degree heart blocks.

Second-Degree Heart Block Type I (Wenckebach, Mobitz Type I) As the sinus node initiates impulses, each one is delayed in the AV node a little longer than the preceding one, until one is eventually blocked completely. Those impulses that are conducted travel normally through the ventricles (Figure 3-7).

REGULARITY: Irregular in a pattern of grouped beating.

RATE: Since some beats are not conducted, the ventricular rate is slower than the atrial rate. The atrial rate is normal.

P-WAVES: Upright and uniform. Some P-waves are not followed by QRS complexes.

PRI: Gets progressively longer, until one P-wave is not followed by a QRS complex. After the blocked beat, the cycle starts again.

QRS: The QRS complex measurement will be normal.

Figure 3-7 Second-Degree AV Block Type I (2° AVB Type I/Wenckebach/Mobitz I)

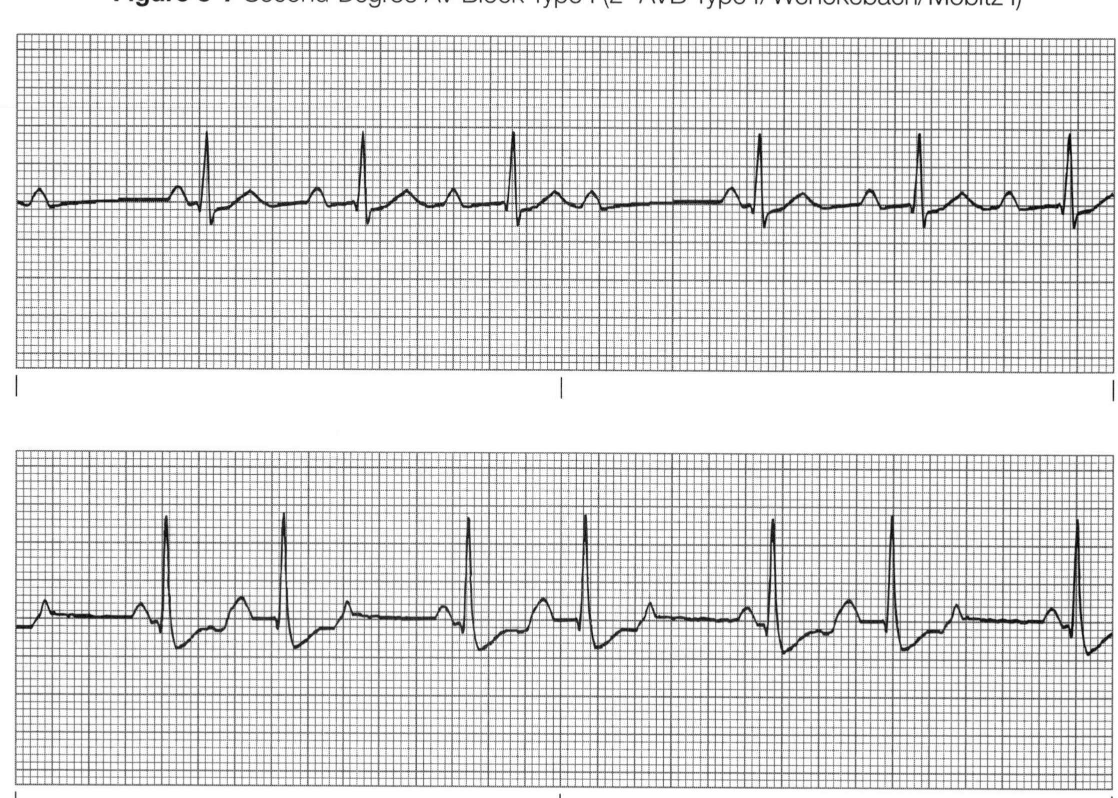

Quick Tip

When you see a heart block, look at the PR interval—"Longer, longer, longer, drop . . . now we have a Wenckebach."

Second-Degree Heart Block Type II (Mobitz Type II) The AV node selectively conducts some beats while blocking others. Those that are not blocked are conducted through to the ventricles. Once in the ventricles, conduction proceeds normally (Figure 3-8).

REGULARITY: If the conduction ratio is consistent, the rhythm will be regular. If the conduction ratio varies, the rhythm will be irregular.

RATE: The atrial rate is usually normal. Since many of the atrial impulses are blocked, the ventricular rate will be lower than the atrial.

P-WAVES: Upright and uniform. There are more P-waves than QRS complexes.

Quick Tip

If you see a heart block, look at the PR interval: "If the PRs look the same to you, then the block's a Mobitz II."

Complete (Third-Degree) Heart Block In complete heart block, the block between the atria and the ventricles is complete. Impulses do not pass

Figure 3-8 Second-Degree AV Block Type II (2° AVB Type II/Mobitz II)

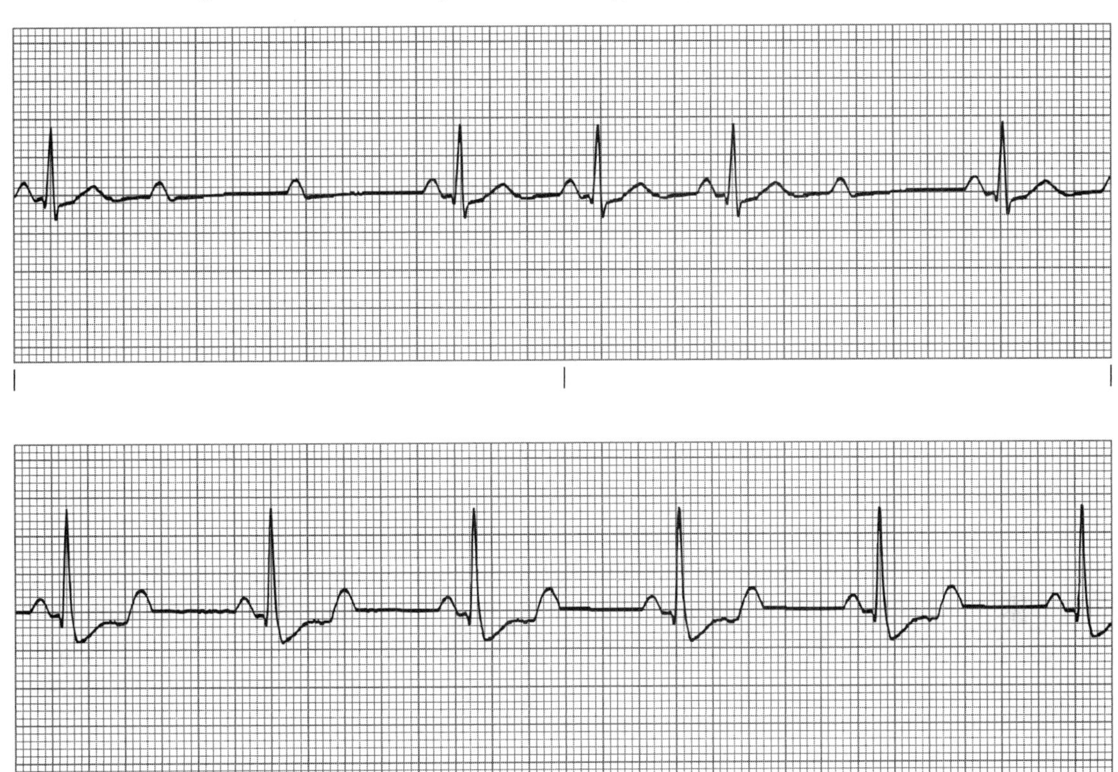

through pathways low in the heart to the ventricles. In the absence of stimulation from above, automatically either the AV junction (if the block is high in the AV node) or the ventricles (if the block is in the bundle branches) will "save the day" and create impulses to depolarize cells low in the heart. The atria and the ventricles function in a totally dissociated fashion—regular P-waves, regular QRS complexes, different rates (Figure 3-9).

REGULARITY: Both the atria and the ventricles are firing so the P-P intervals and the R-R intervals will be regular.

RATE: The atrial rate will usually be in a normal range. The ventricular rate may be 20–60.

P-WAVES: More P-waves than QRS complexes.

PRI: No atrial impulses conducted to the ventricles. The P-waves have no relationship to the QRS complexes. A P-wave may occasionally be found on or near a QRS complex, but no patter to the PR intervals can be found.

QRS: If the ventricles are being controlled by a junctional focus, the QRS complex will measure less than 0.12 seconds. If the focus is ventricular the QRS will be wide.

Figure 3-9 Third-Degree AV Block (3° AVB/Complete Heart Block)

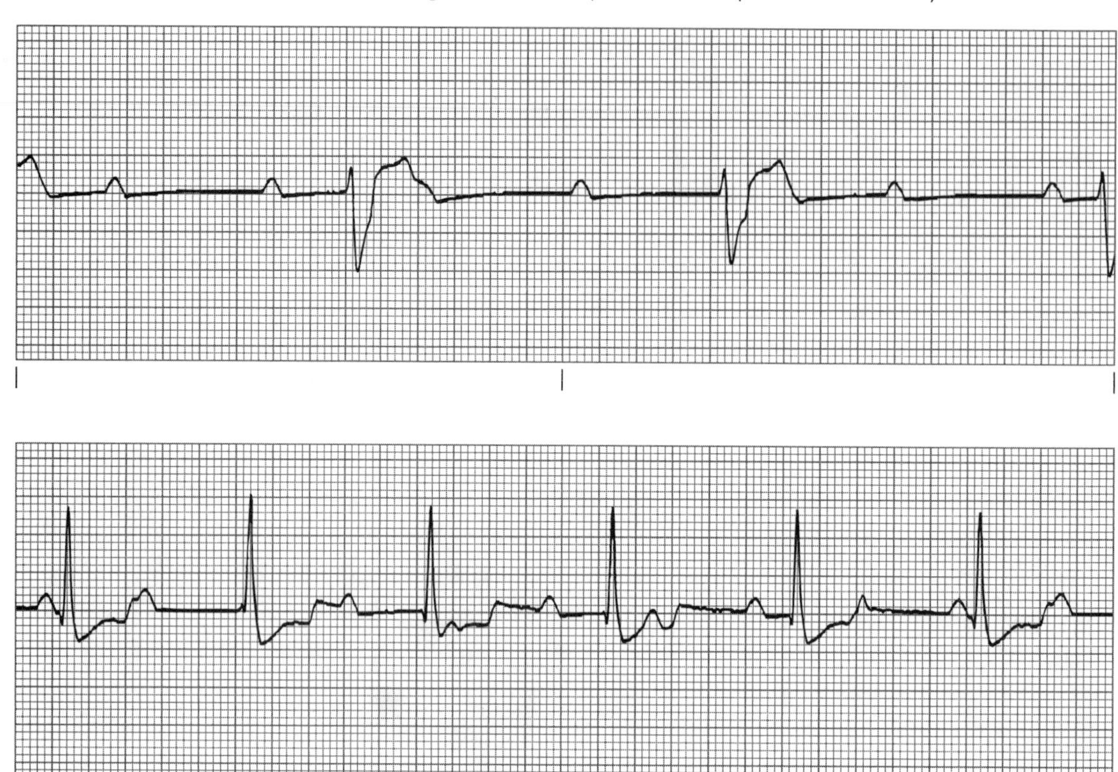

Quick Tip

If you see a heart block, look at the PR interval. "If the PRs make no sense to thee, then you have a third-degree."

TACHYCARDIAS

Tachycardias concern us in ACLS because fast heart rates create high oxygen demand for the myocardium, putting the patient at risk for ischemic events if his coronary arteries are narrowed. In addition, stroke volume, or the amount of blood that is ejected with each heartbeat, is partially dependent on the amount of blood in the ventricles at the time of contraction. With rapid heart rates, the time allowed for the ventricles to fill is very short, potentially decreasing the amount of blood that can be ejected when the ventricles contract. Tachycardia is not a state that we'd like to continue in our patients for very long, no matter how they are feeling.

Tachycardia generally means "fast rate." We must further classify tachycardias as either wide or narrow (referring to the width of the QRS complex) and stable or unstable (referring to the patient status. Unless you have information to the contrary:

- Consider wide rhythms to be ventricular in origin.
- Consider narrow rhythms to be supraventricular in origin.

Supraventricular Tachycardia

Supraventricular is a geographic term that describes rhythms that originate above (supra) the ventricles in the heart. This can include atrial tachycardias, atrial fibrillation, or atrial flutter with ventricular responses greater than 150 per minute, junctional tachycardias, and a variety of other unusual rhythms.

Figure 3-10 Atrial tachycardia (A-tach)

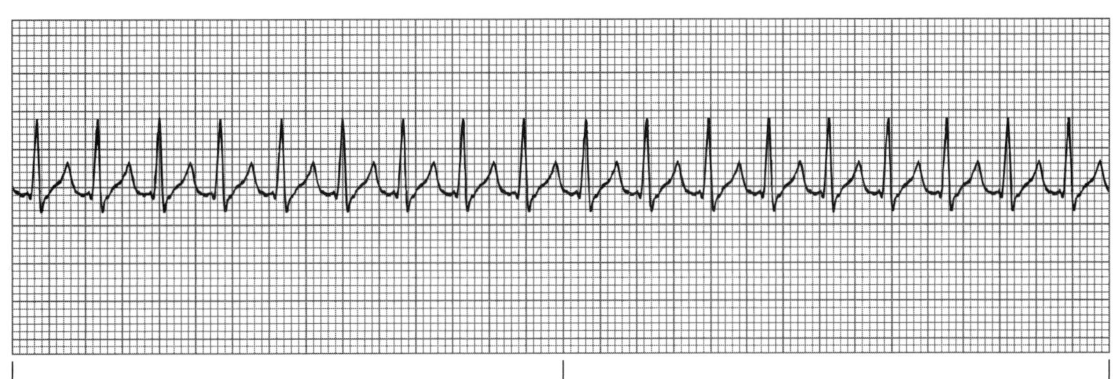

Generally speaking, the hallmarks of supraventricular tachycardias are the rate greater than 150 per minute and the narrow (normal) width of the QRS complexes. Some rhythms that may result in supraventricular tachycardia include:

Atrial Tachycardia. The pacemaker is a single irritable site within the atrium, which fires repetitively at a very rapid rate. Conduction through the ventricles is normal (Figure 3-10).

REGULARITY:	Regular.
RATE:	Usually 150–250.
P-WAVES:	There is one P-wave for every QRS but it is usually hidden in the T-wave. As the P-wave and the T-wave come together they make a peak between the complexes.
PRI:	Normal, not measurable if the P-wave is hidden in the T-wave.
QRS:	Within normal limits.

Quick Tip

If the rate is fast and you see "teepees" (pointy T-waves that may have P-waves buried within) think "atrial tachycardia."

Atrial Flutter. A single irritable focus within the atria generates impulses that are conducted in a rapid, repetitive fashion. To protect the ventricles from receiving too many impulses, the AV node blocks some of the impulses from being conducted through to the ventricles (Figure 3-11).

REGULARITY:	May be regular or irregular depending on conduction pattern.
RATE:	Atrial rate is 250–350 beats per minute. Ventricular rate may range from normal to severe tachycardia.
P-WAVES:	In atrial flutter produce a sawtooth appearance.
PRI:	Because of the unusual configuration of the flutter wave and the proximity of the wave to the QRS complex, it is often impossible to determine a PRI. Therefore, the PRI is not measured.
QRS:	Within normal limits.

Quick Tip

The baseline of this rhythm (the area between the QRS complexes) often looks like a saw. Think "flutter-cutter."

Figure 3-11 Atrial flutter

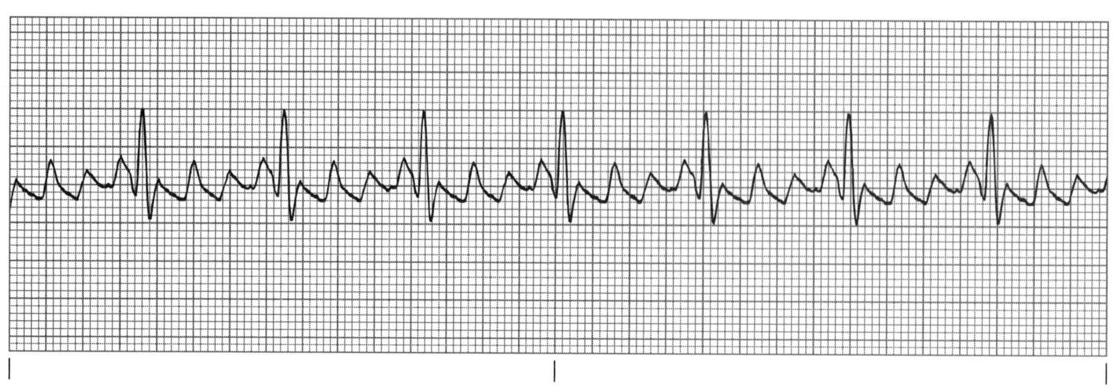

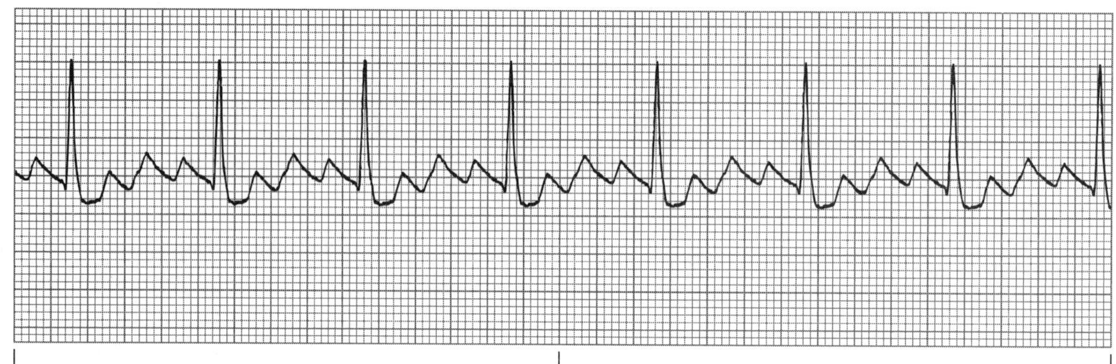

Atrial Fibrillation. The atria are so irritable that they rapidly initiate impulses, causing the atria to depolarize repeatedly in a fibrillatory manner. The AV node blocks most of the impulses, allowing only a limited number through to the ventricles (Figure 3-12).

REGULARITY: The ventricular rate is grossly irregular.

RATE: The atrial rate cannot be measured because it is over 300 per minute. The ventricular rate may range from bradycardia to severe tachycardia, depending on how many impulses are conducted by the AV node down to the ventricles.

P-WAVES: The rapid atrial firing creates a wavy fibrillatory wave where the P-wave is normally found.

PRI: Since individual P waves are not visible, the PR interval cannot be measured.

QRS: Usually narrow (within normal limits).

Quick Tip

Remember that the baseline of this rhythm (the area between the QRS complexes) is undulating, bumpy, and erratic. Think "fibble-scribble."

Clinical Note: For ACLS, the biggest concern about atrial fibrillation and atrial flutter

Figure 3-12 Atrial fibrillation

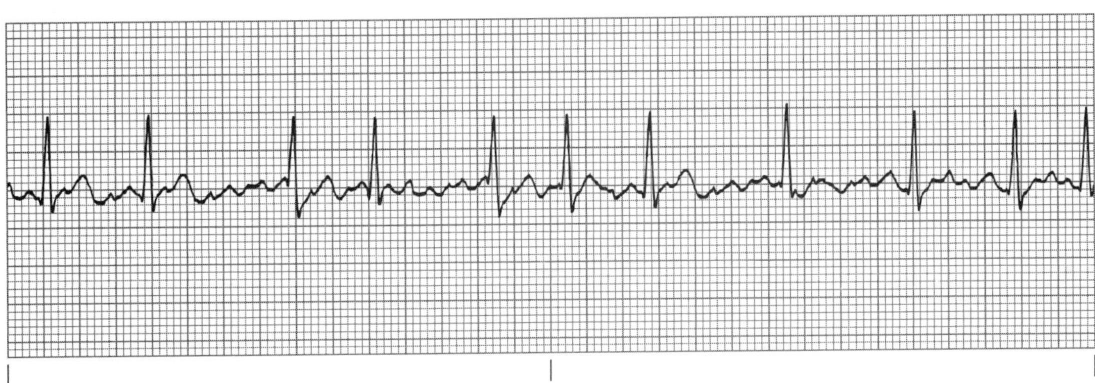

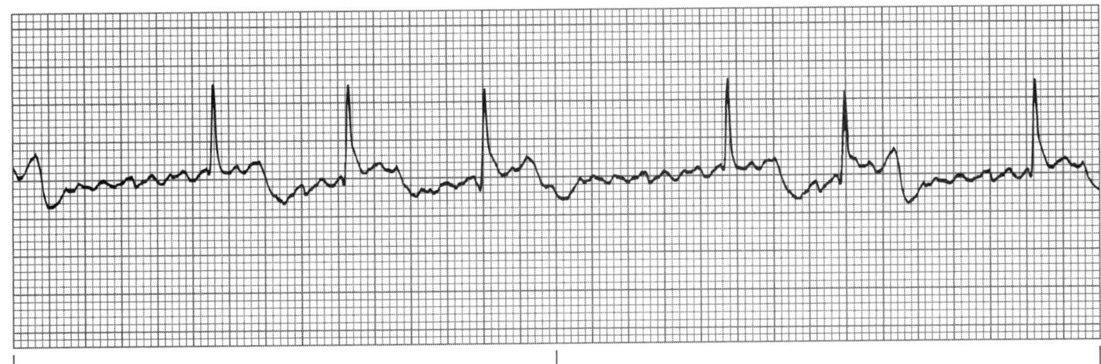

is whether the rate is well controlled. If the patient is tachycardic, the initial goal should be to control the rate, rather than convert to another rhythm. Patients in atrial fibrillation for more than 48 hours are at risk for clots forming in their atria as a result of stagnant blood. If the rhythm is converted to one with organized atrial contraction, there is a possibility that embolic events could occur.

Ventricular Tachycardia

An irritable focus in the ventricles fires regularly at a rate greater than 100 times per minute to override other pacemakers for control of the heart (Figure 3-13).

REGULARITY: Regular.
RATE: Atrial rate cannot be determined. Ventricular rate exceeds 100.
P-WAVES: P-waves are difficult to visualize.
PRI: PR interval cannot be measured if P-waves cannot be identified.
QRS: Wide (>0.12 seconds) and bizarre.

Other Ventricular Rhythms

Ventricular Ectopy. Ventricular ectopic beats are a sign of an irritable myocardium. They can be treated if they cause hemodynamic instability, but the goal for patient therapy is to find and treat the cause of the irritability.

PVCs, or premature ventricular contractions, are wide, look different from the patient's "normal" beats, and occur early, making the rhythm irregular. PVCs that all look the same come from

Figure 3-13 Ventricular tachycardia

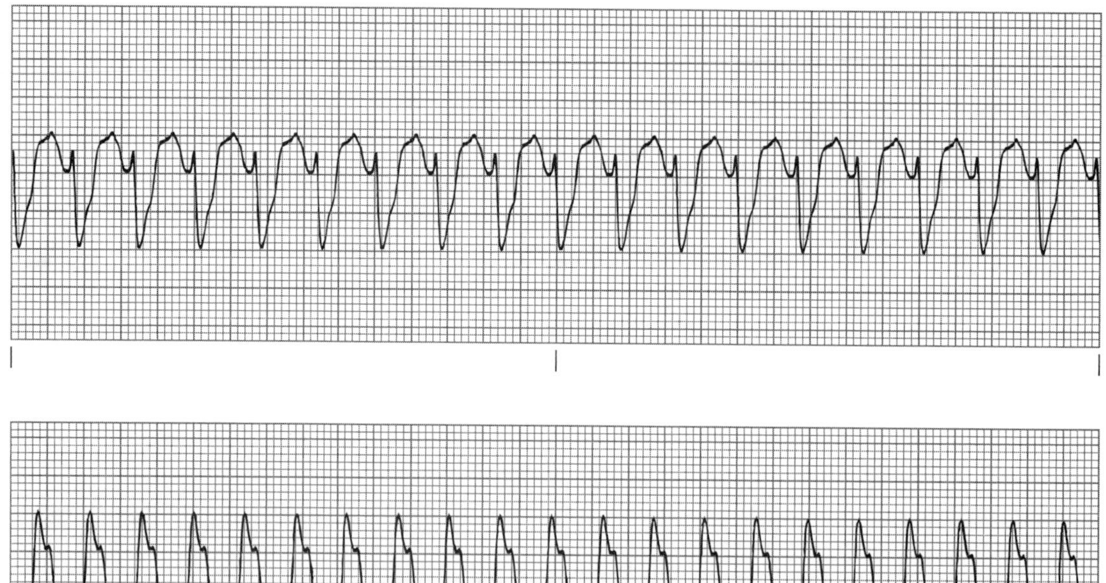

the same focus in the heart and are called *unifocal* (Figure 3-14). PVCs that look different from each other are from different foci and are called *multifocal* (Figure 3-15). Ventricular beats may occur in groups of two (pairs or couplets) or three (salvos) (Figure 3-16). The underlying rhythm should be identified in addition to describing the PVCs.

Ventricular Fibrillation. The most common arrhythmia found in the adult cardiac arrest victim, ventricular fibrillation is converted to a

Figure 3-14 Normal sinus rhythm with unifocal PVCs

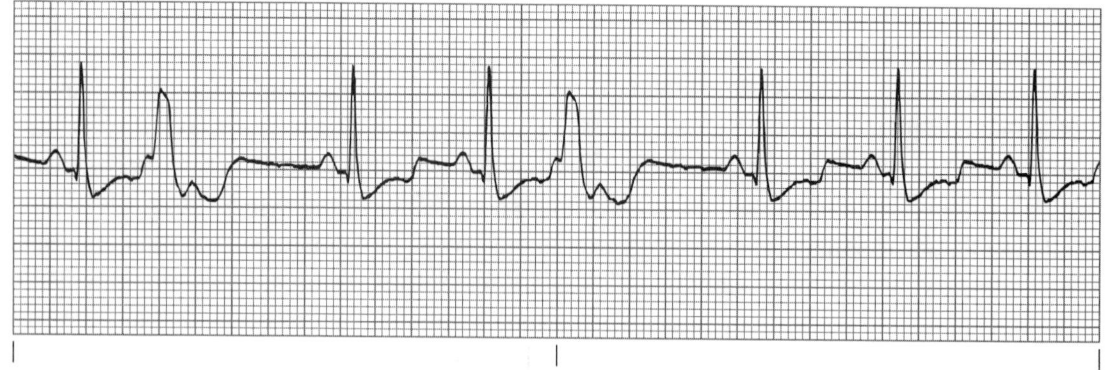

Figure 3-15 Normal sinus rhythm with multifocal PVCs

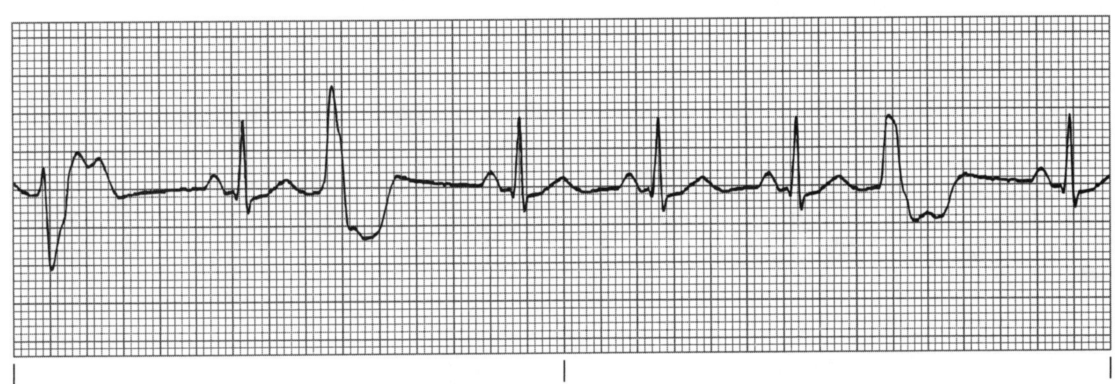

perfusing rhythm only by defibrillation. The heart muscle is in a state of electrical chaos with no pumping action. Without pumping, there is no pulse (Figure 3-17).

REGULARITY:	No waves or complexes. Chaotic.
RATE:	Cannot be determined.
P-WAVES:	No discernible P-waves.
PRI:	No PRI.
QRS:	No discernible QRS complexes.

Asystole

Asystole is the absence of electrical activity. Without electrical activity, there is no mechanical activity, or pumping, of the heart. Few patients who progress to asystole for more than a minute or two will be resuscitated (Figure 3-18).

REGULARITY:	Flat line.
RATE:	Flat line.
P-WAVES:	None, flat line.
PRI:	Flat line.
QRS:	Flat line.

Quick Tip

When you see asystole, the first step is to confirm that there really is absence of electrical activity. Assess the patient, check to see that electrodes are in place, cables are connected, check to be sure the "gain" or ECG size has not been turned down, and look at the rhythm in another lead on your cardiac monitor.

Figure 3-16 Normal sinus rhythm with pairs/couplet PVCs

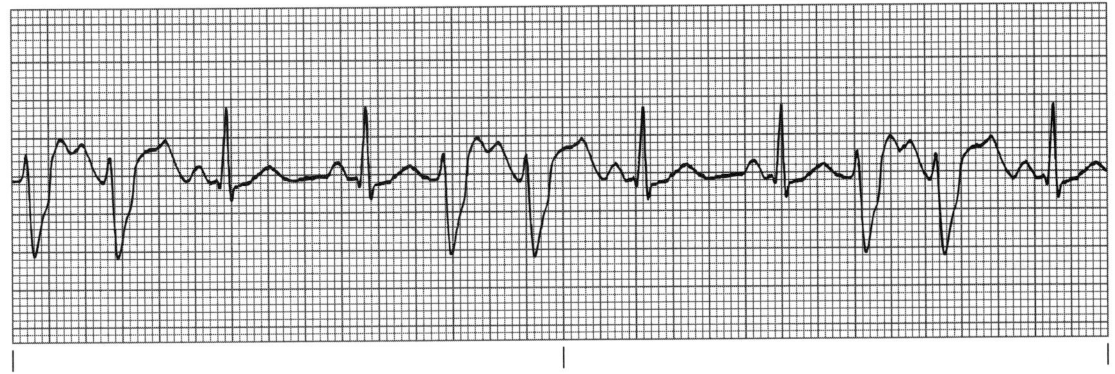

Figure 3-17 Ventricular fibrillation

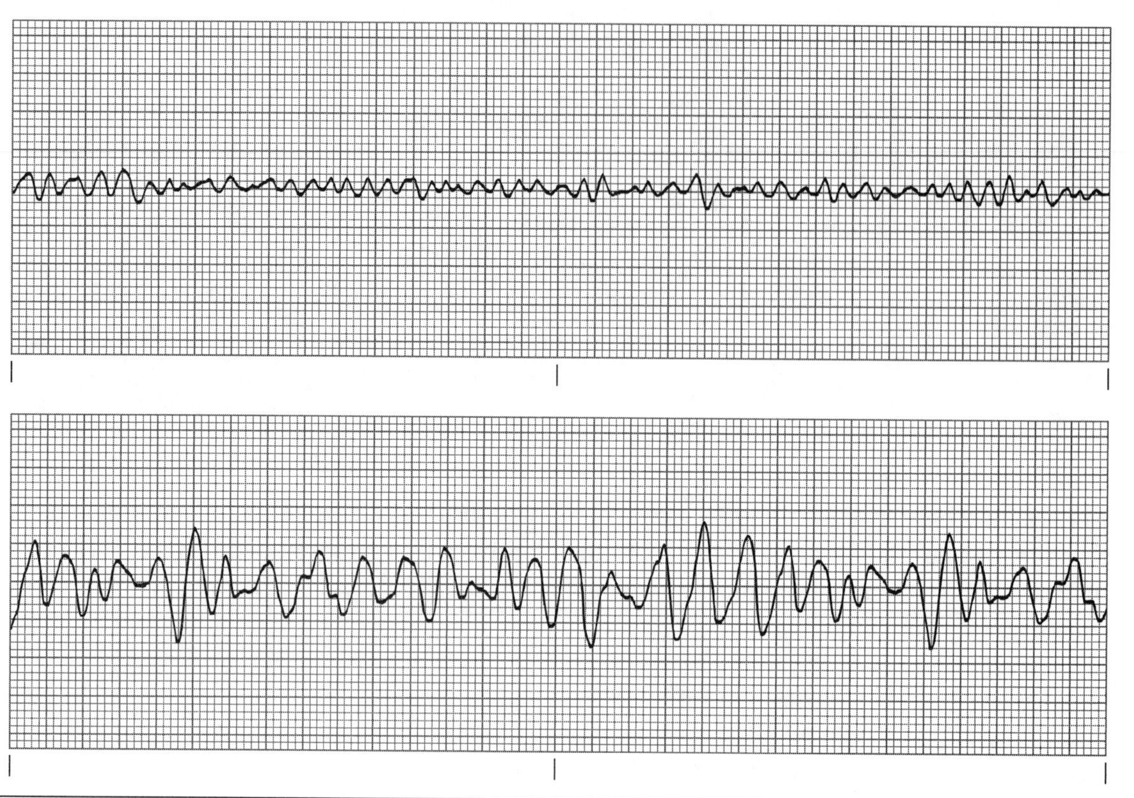

Figure 3-18 Asystole

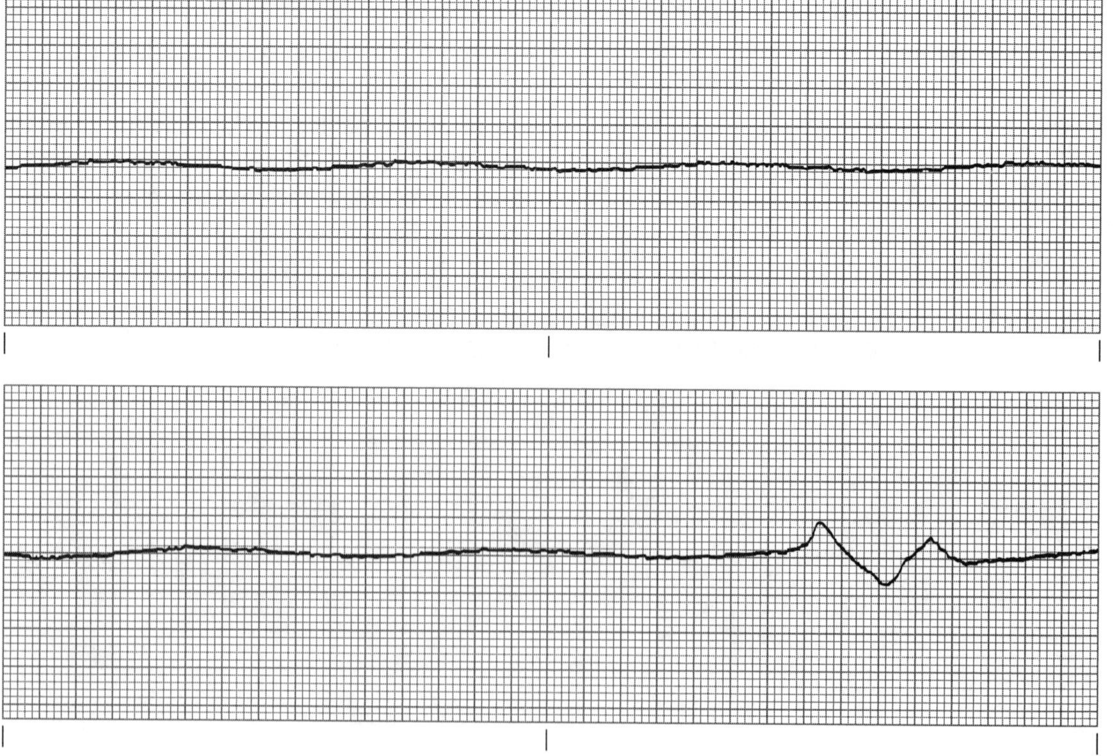

Figure 3-19 Pacemaker in capture

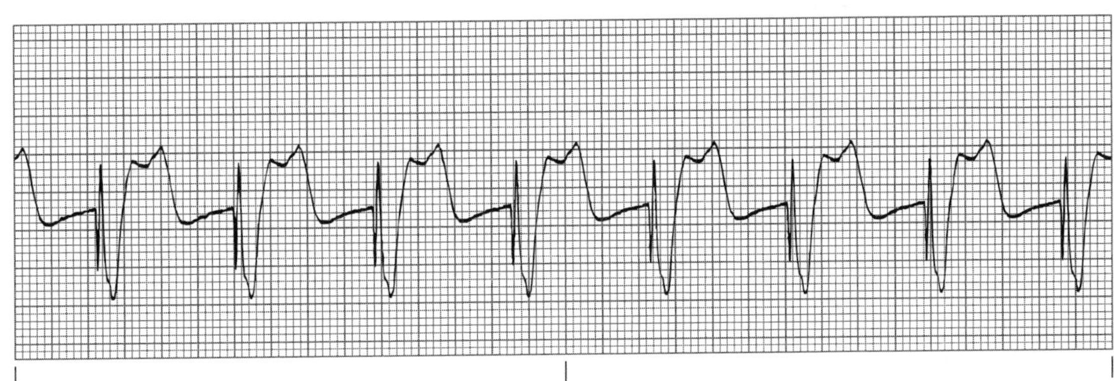

Pacemaker Rhythms

When a pacemaker fires, a vertical "spike" is produced on the monitor. Each spike should be followed by a complex (a P-wave for atrial pacemakers, a QRS complex for ventricular pacemakers). For pacing to be effective, each complex should correspond with a pulse in the patient (Figure 3-19).

Practice Test 1 Identifying Rhythms

Name the following cardiac rhythms:

1.

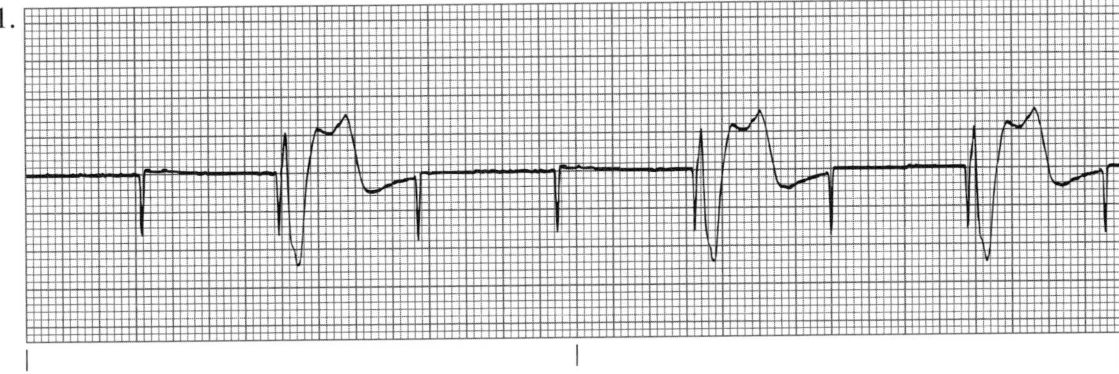

2.

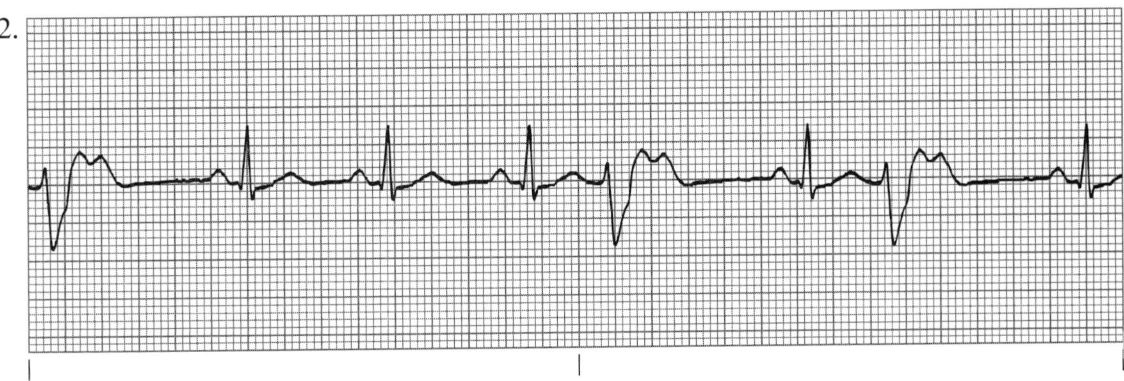

3.

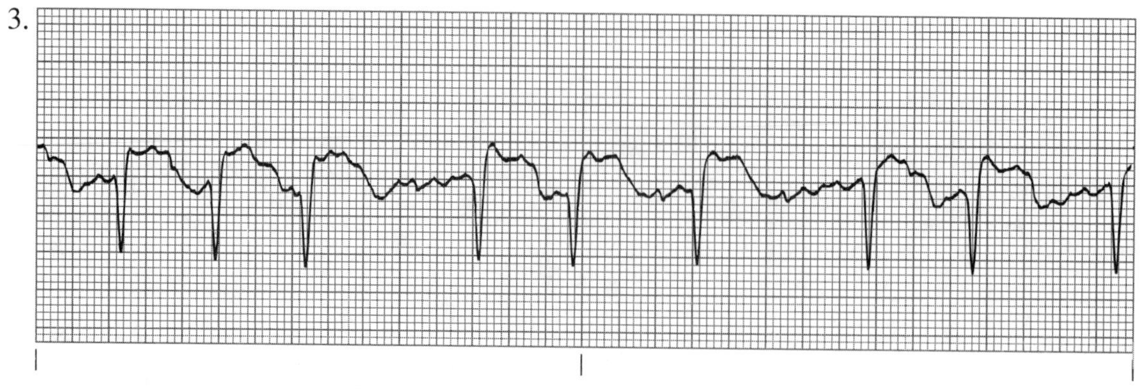

4.

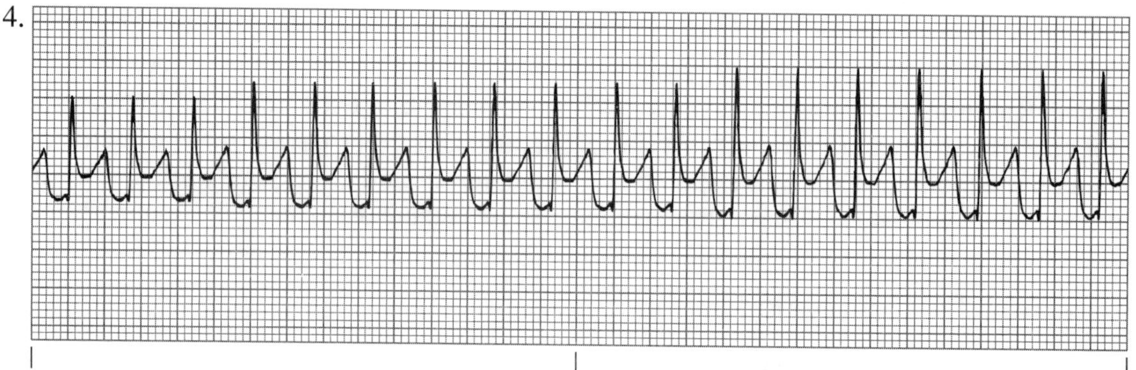

5.

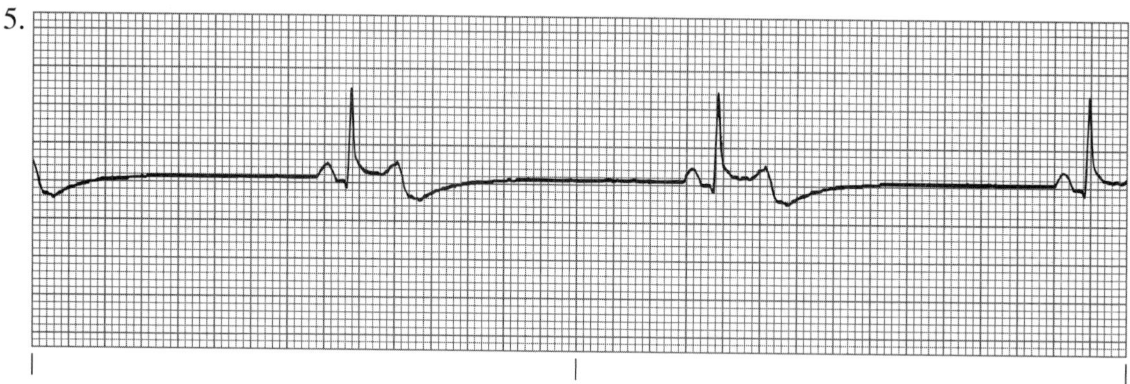

6.

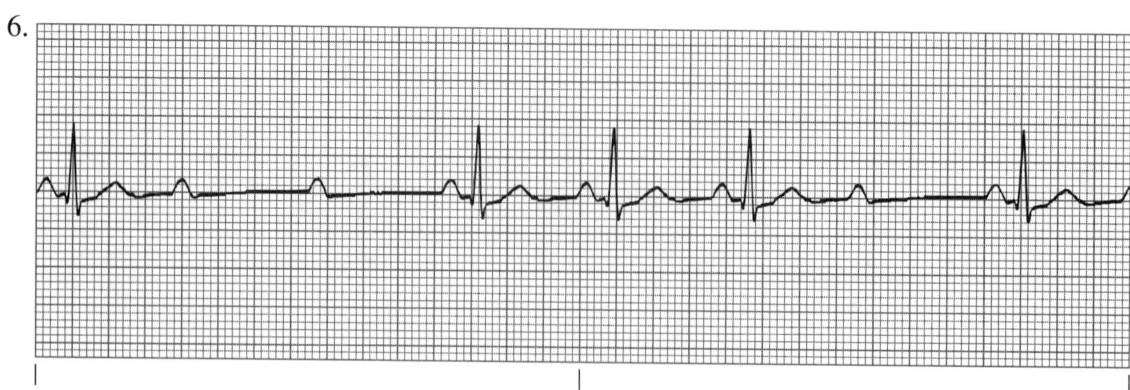

7.

8.

9.

10.

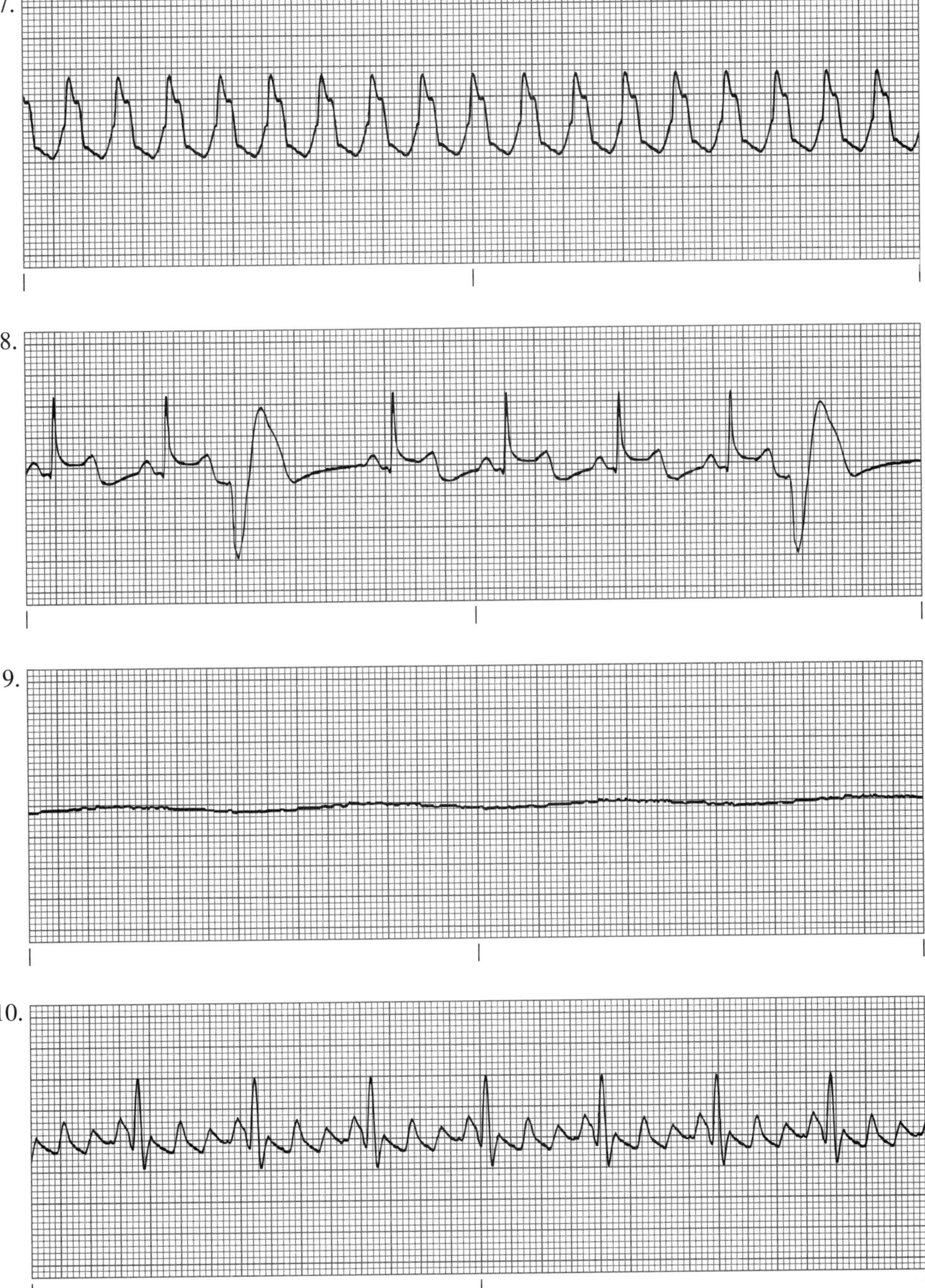

11.

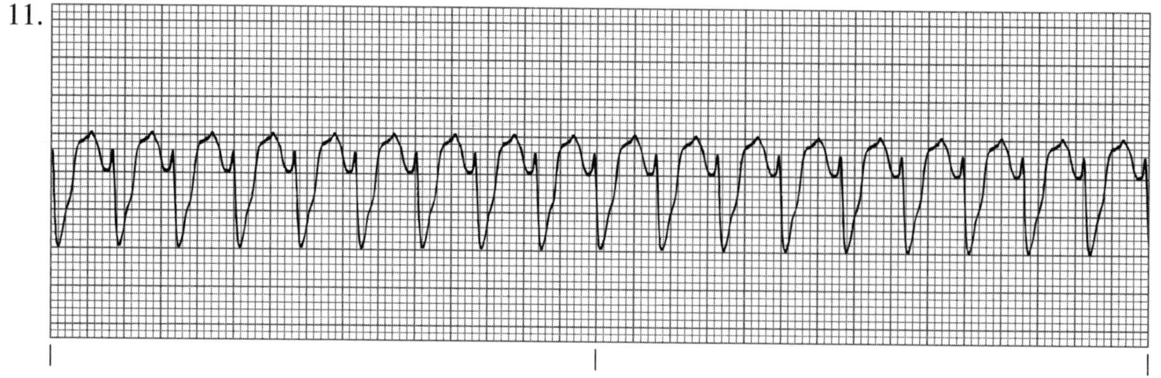

12.

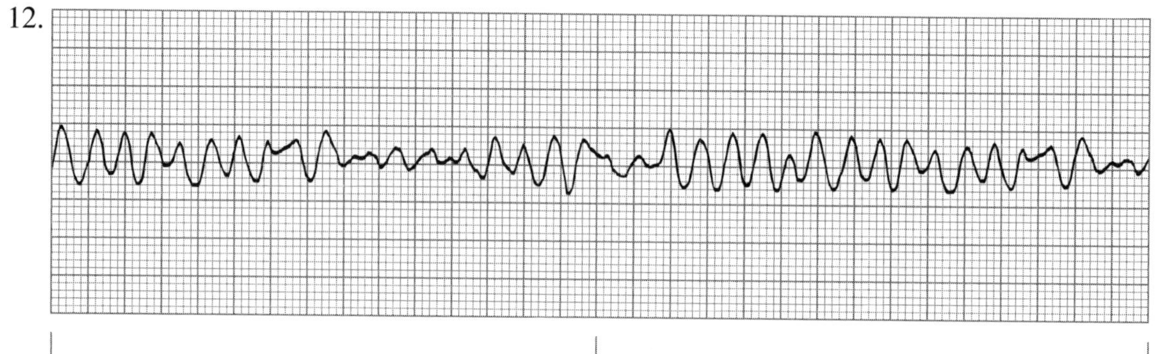

13.

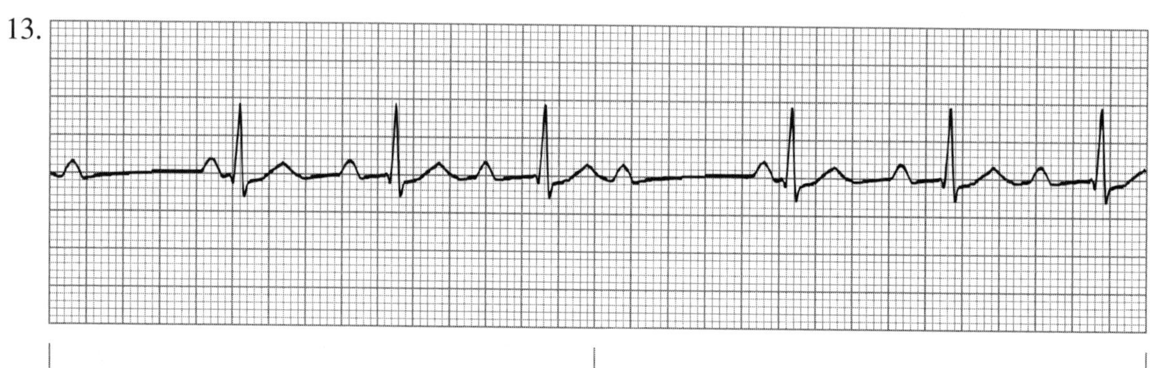

14.

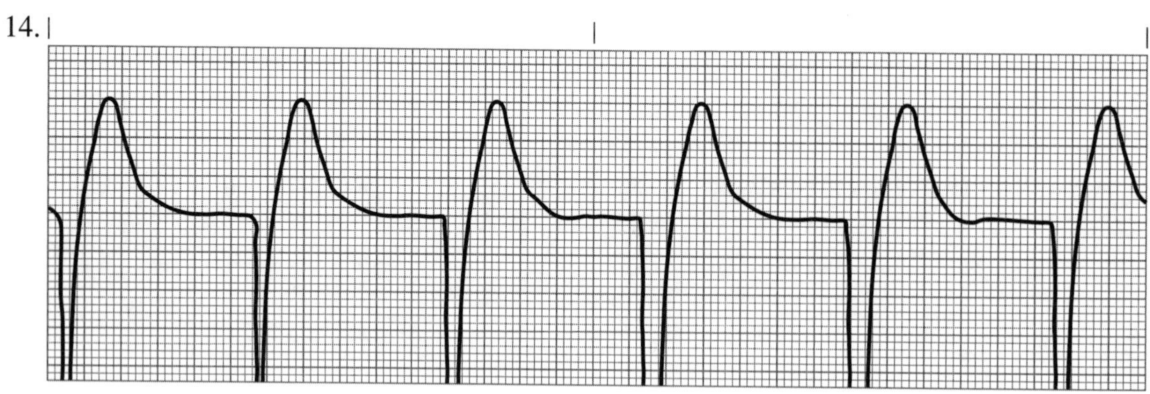

15.

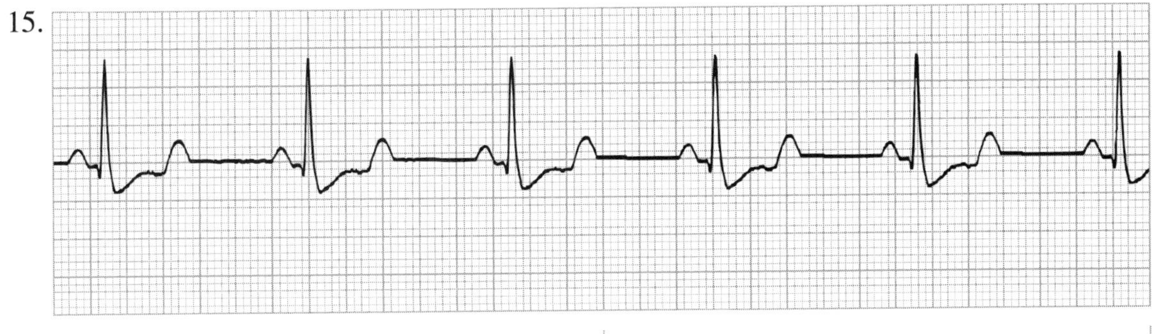

16.

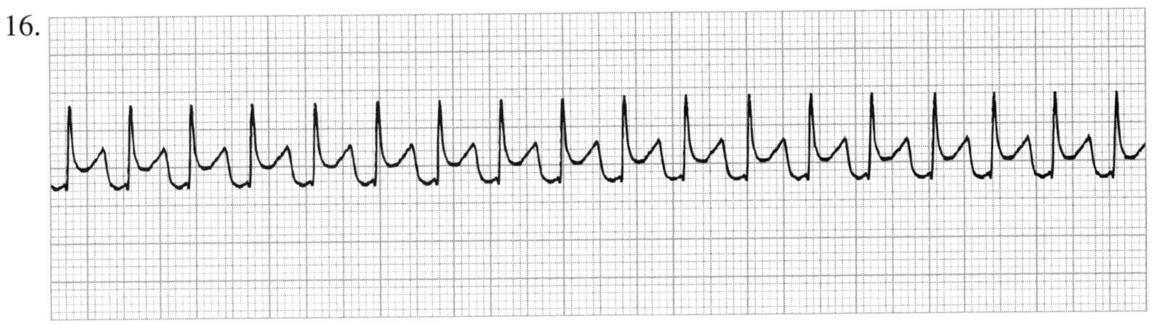

17.

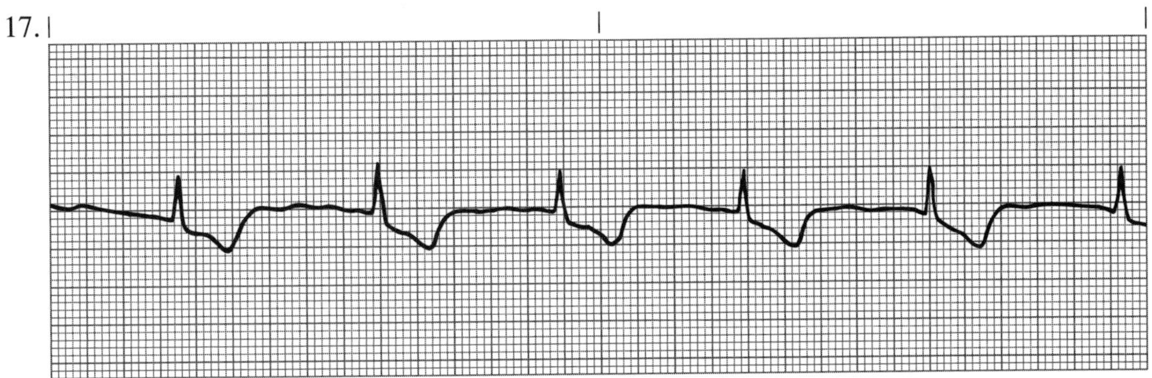

18.

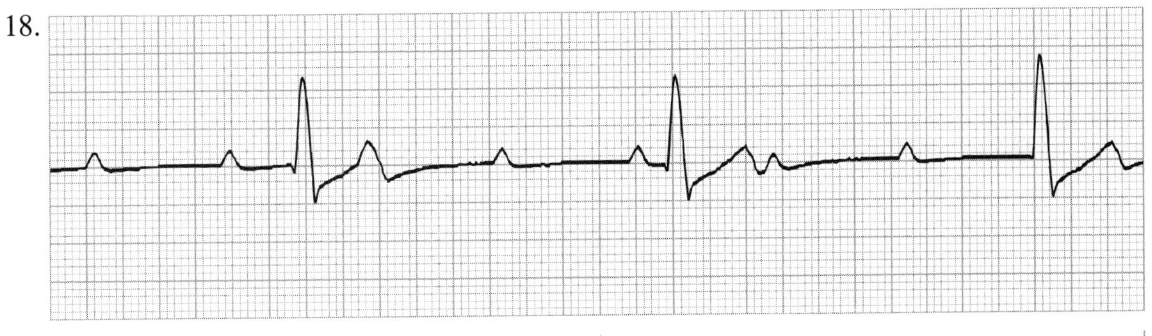

19.

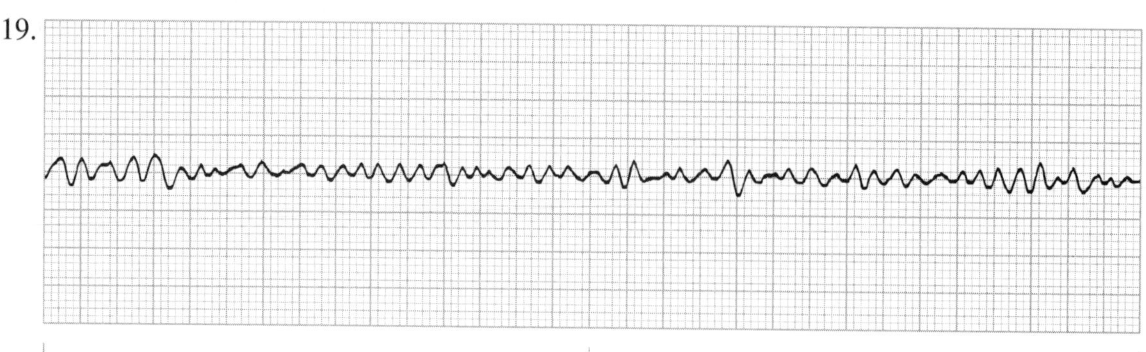

20.

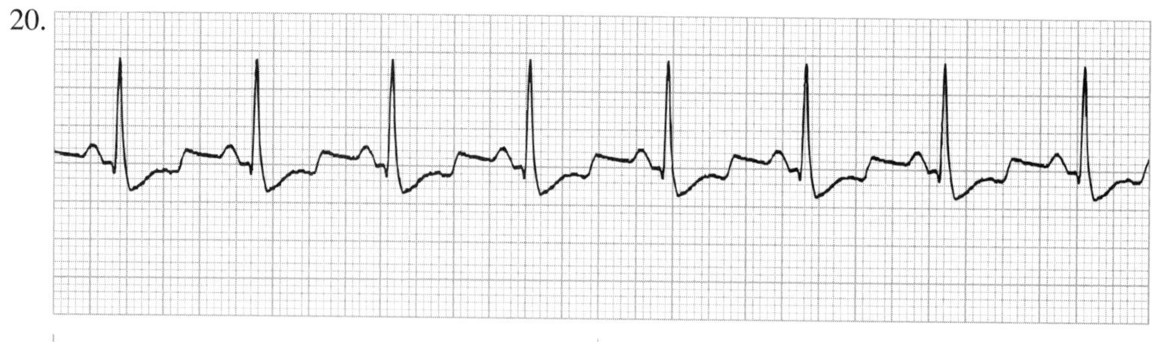

21.

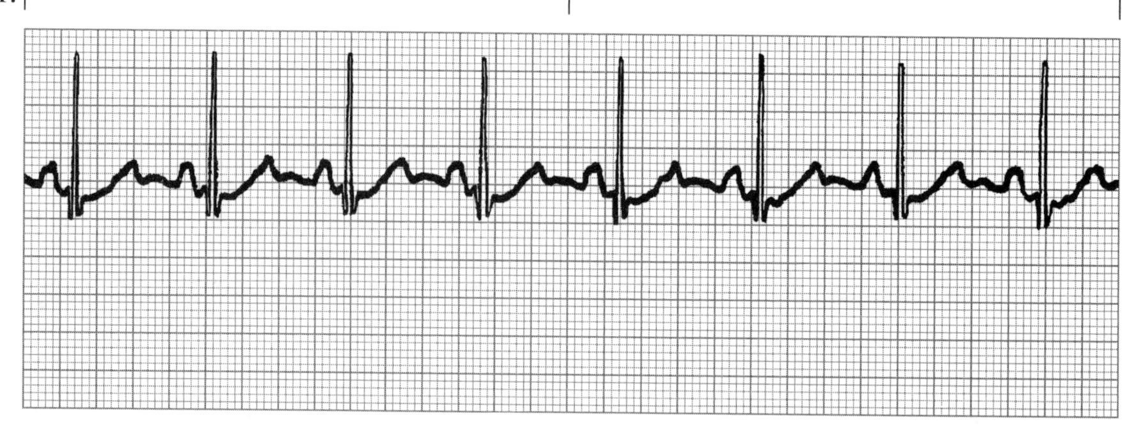

22.

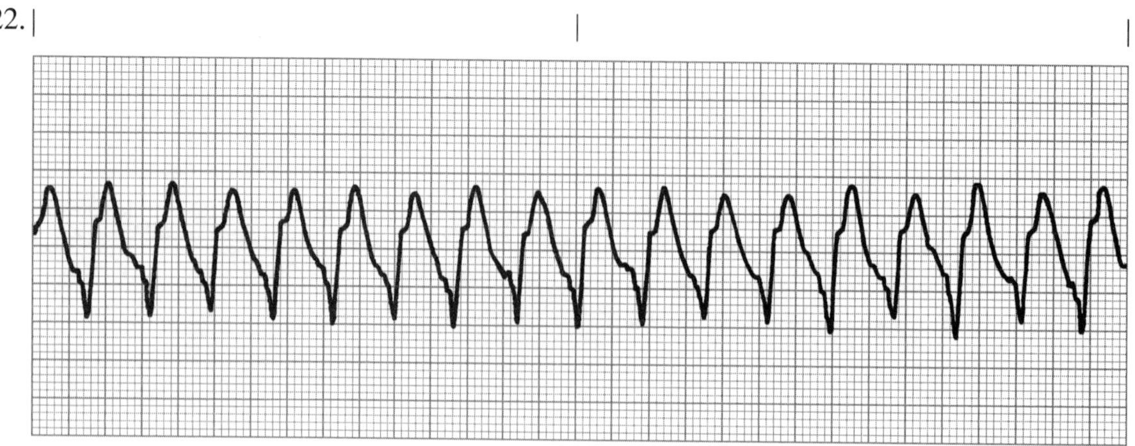

23.

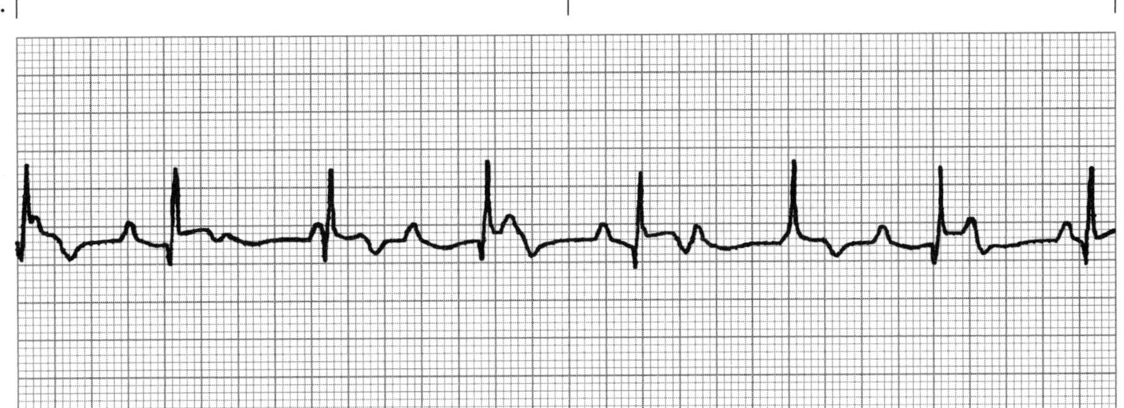

24.

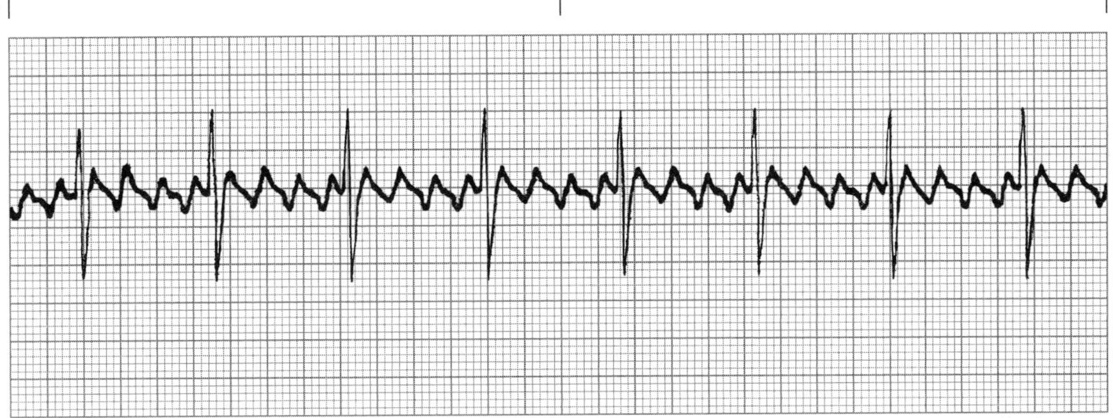

25.

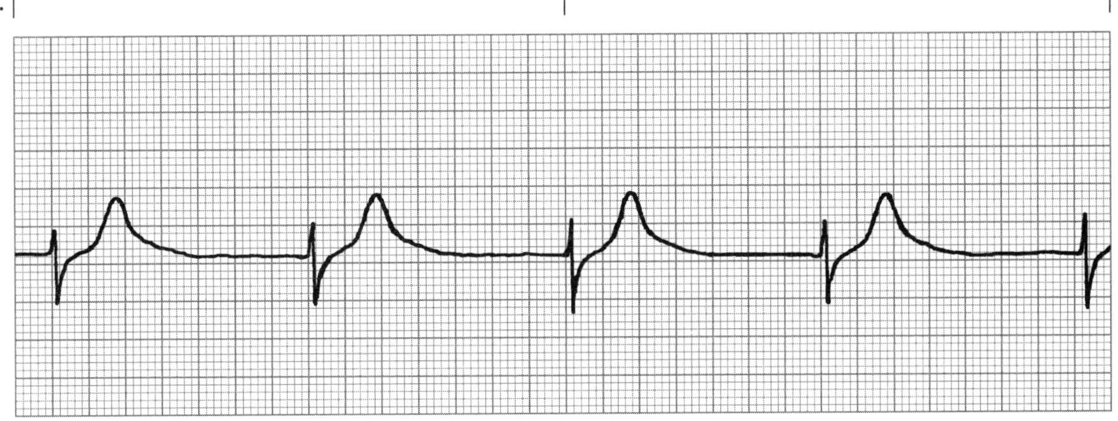

26.
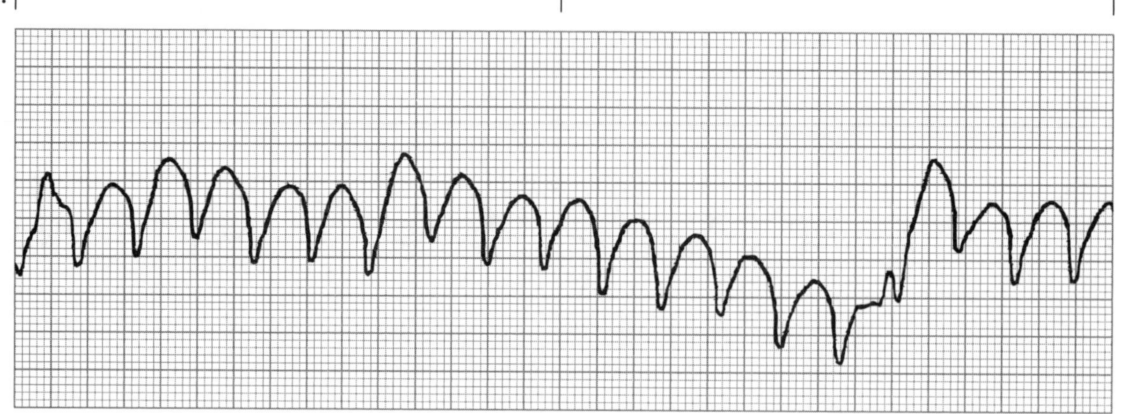

27.
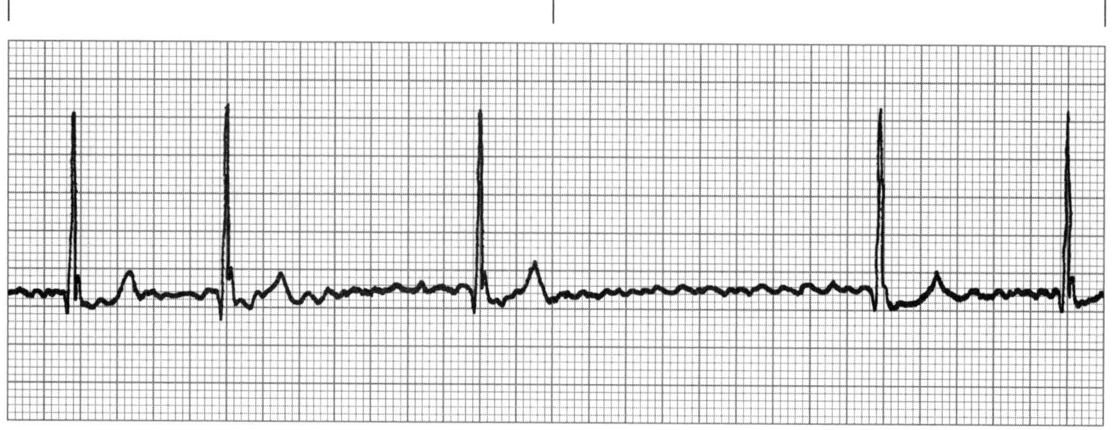

28.
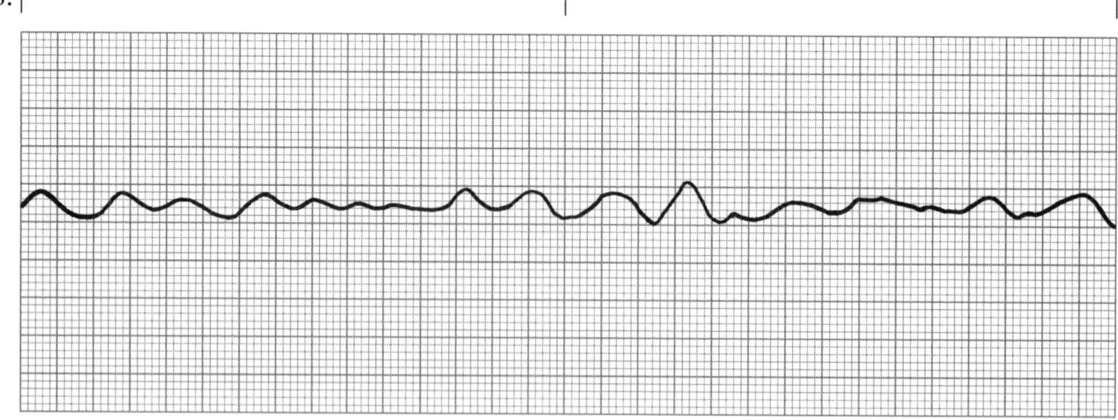

29.

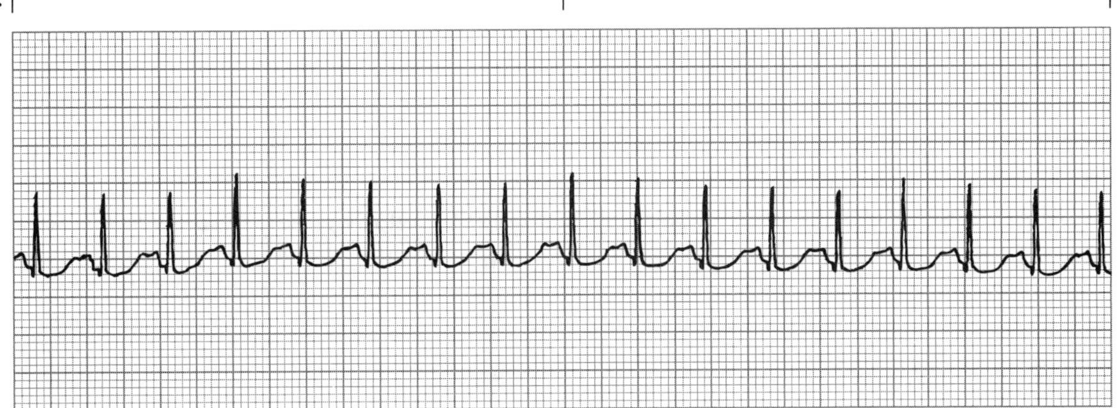

30.

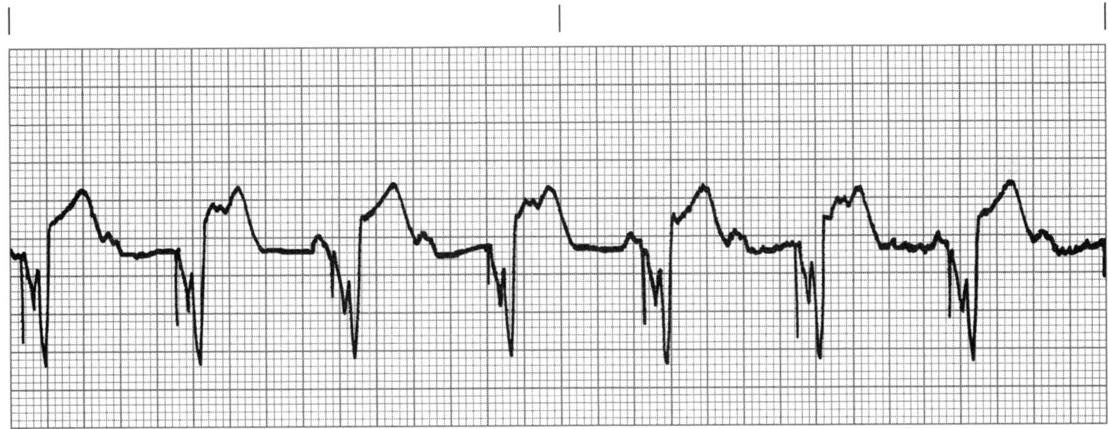

31.

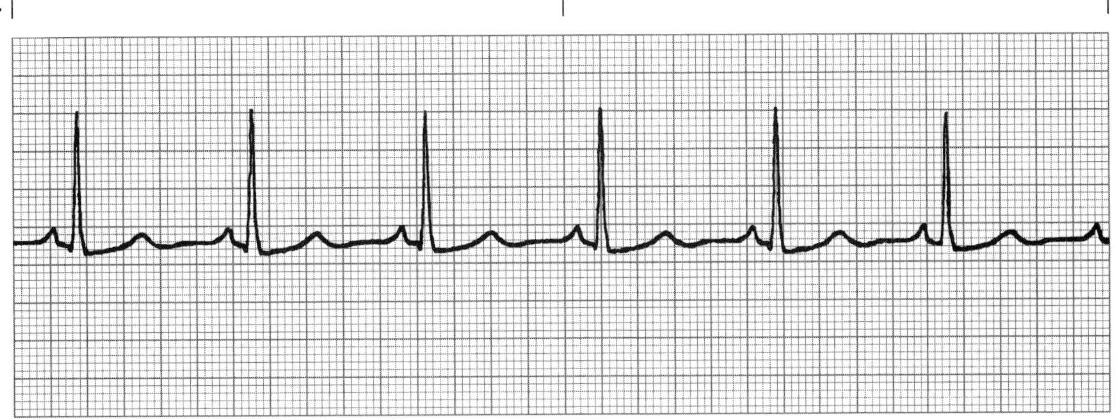

32.

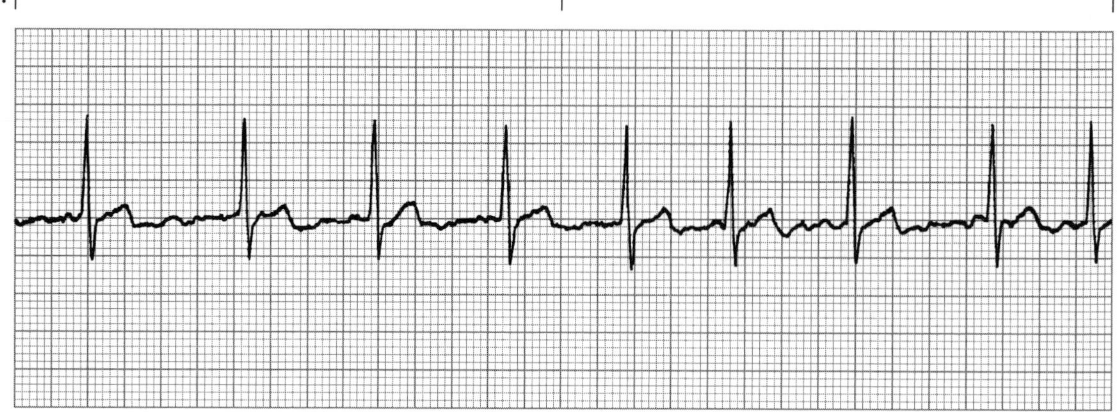

33.

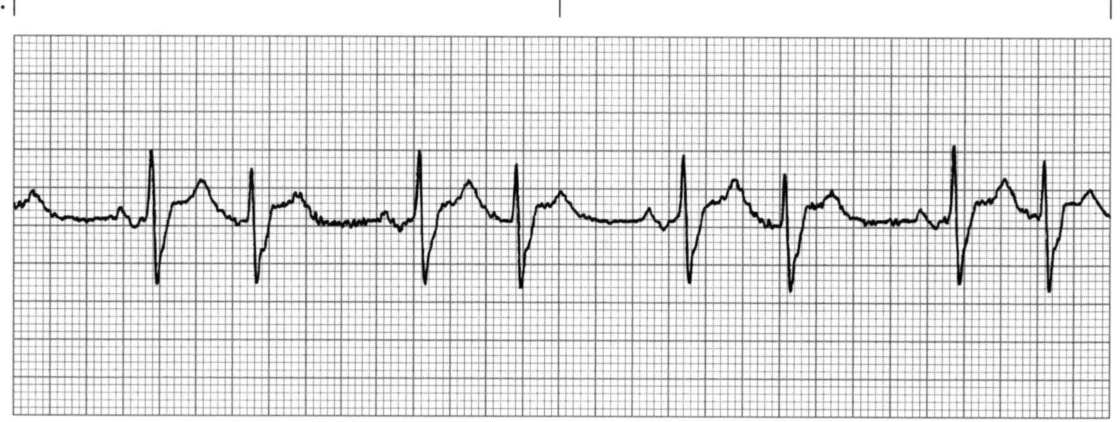

34.

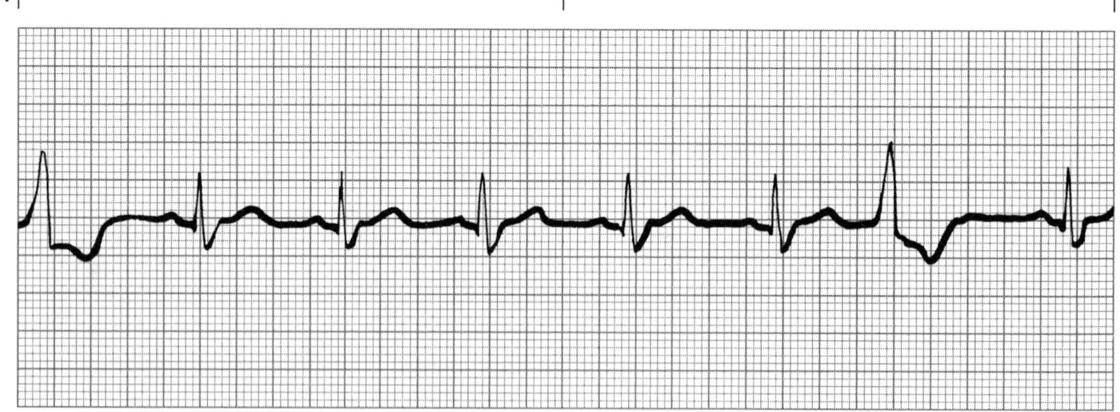

35.

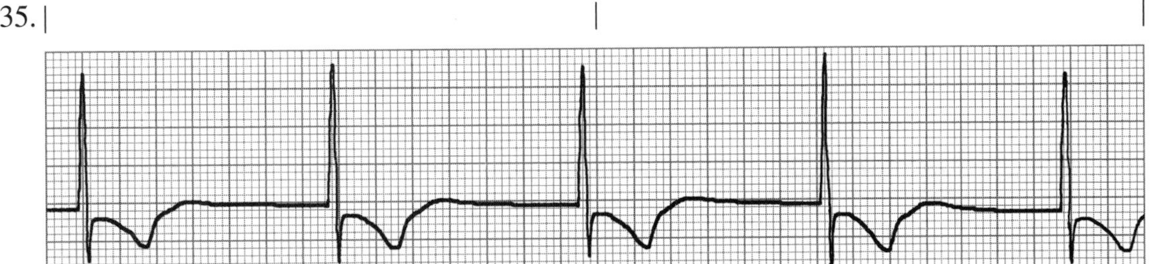

36.

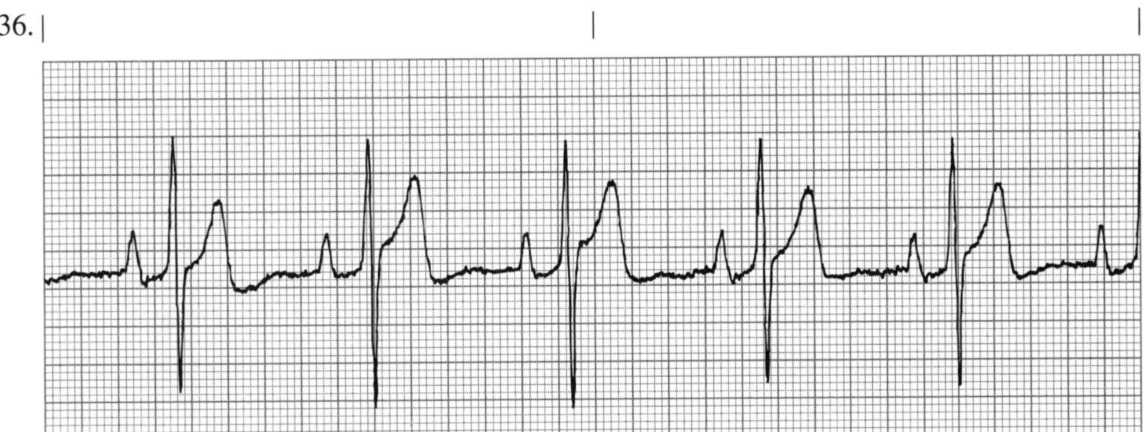

37.

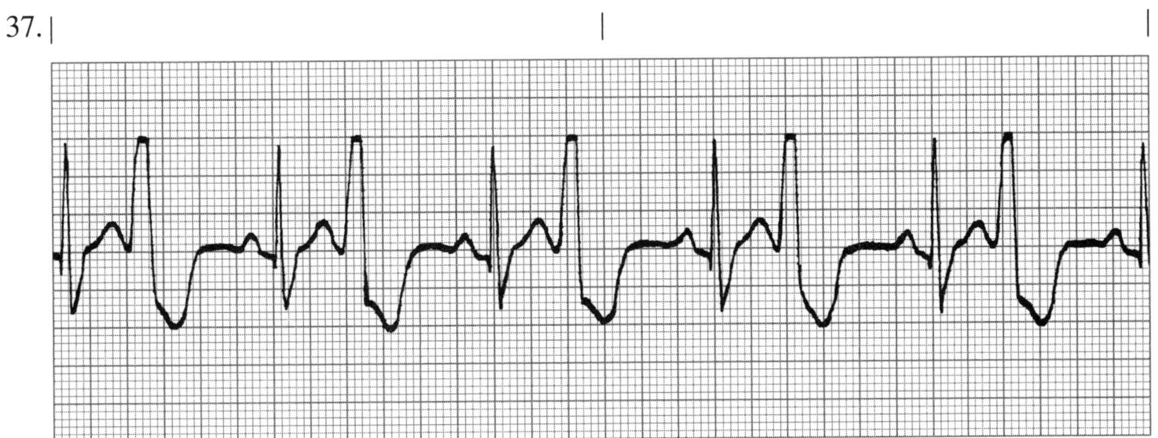

38.

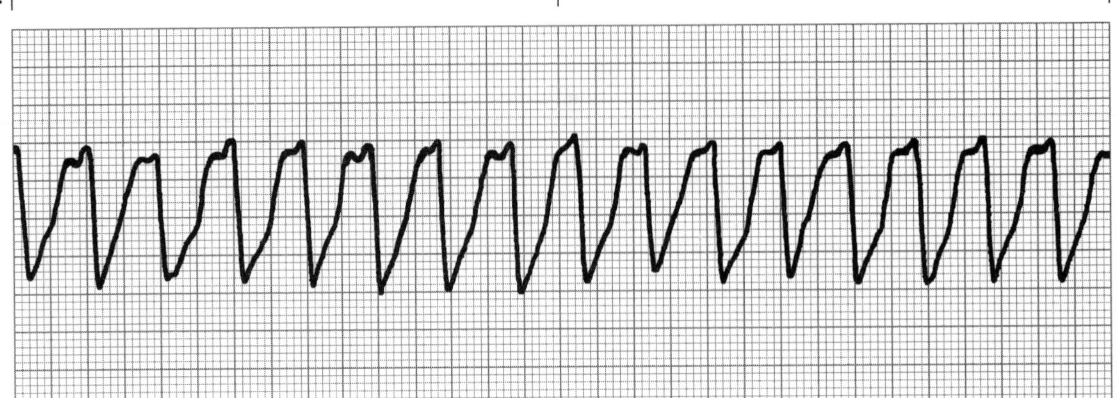

39.

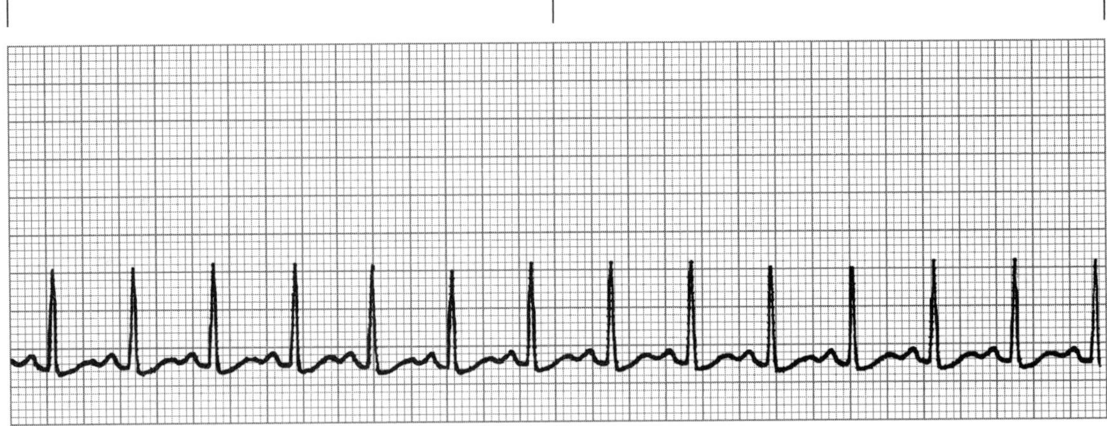

40.

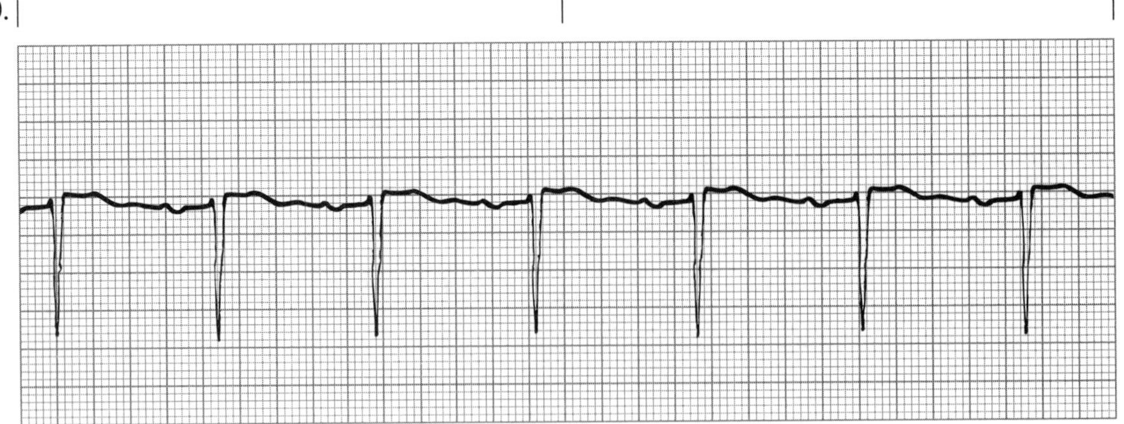

41.

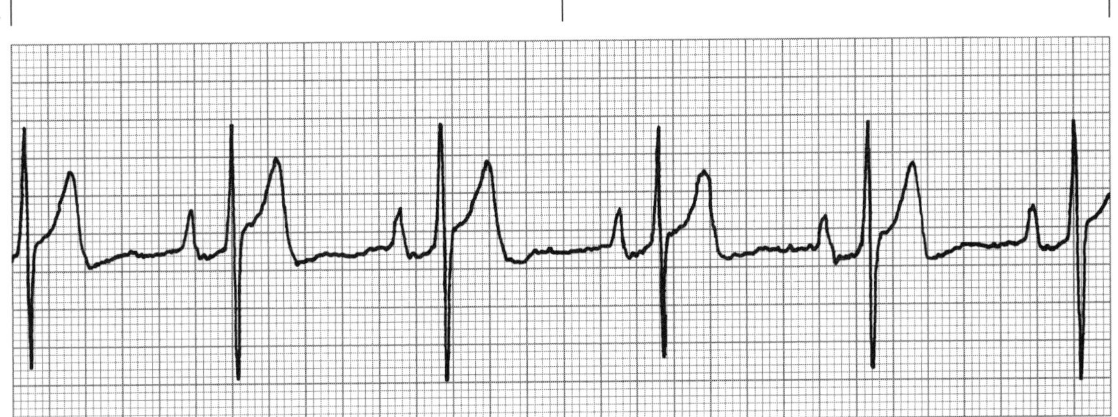

42.

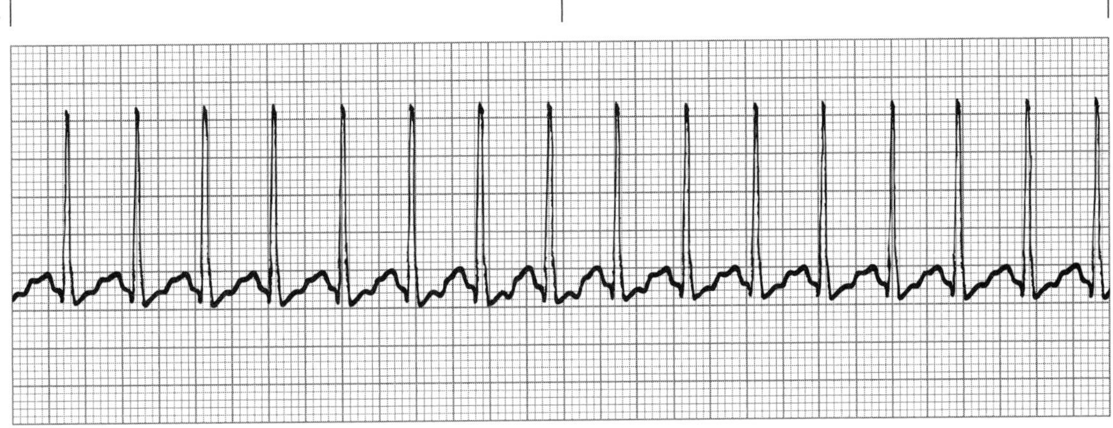

43.

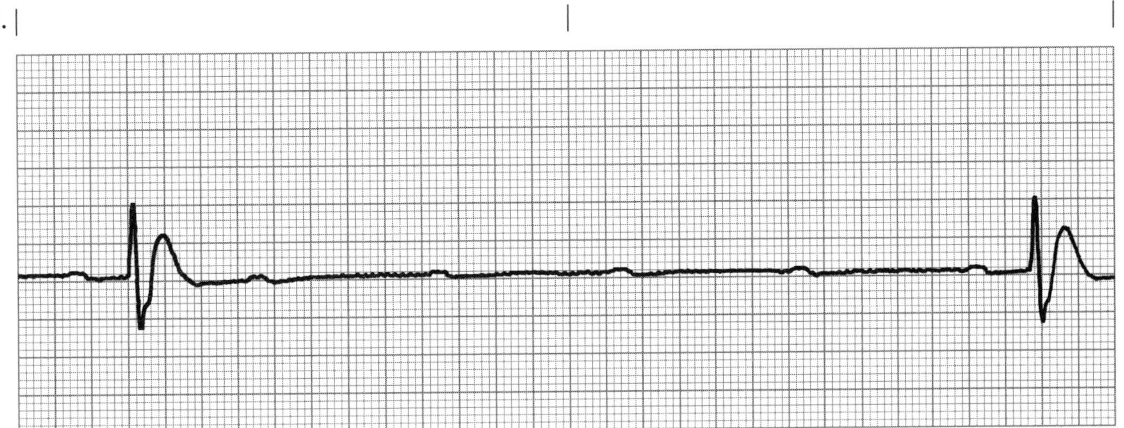

44.

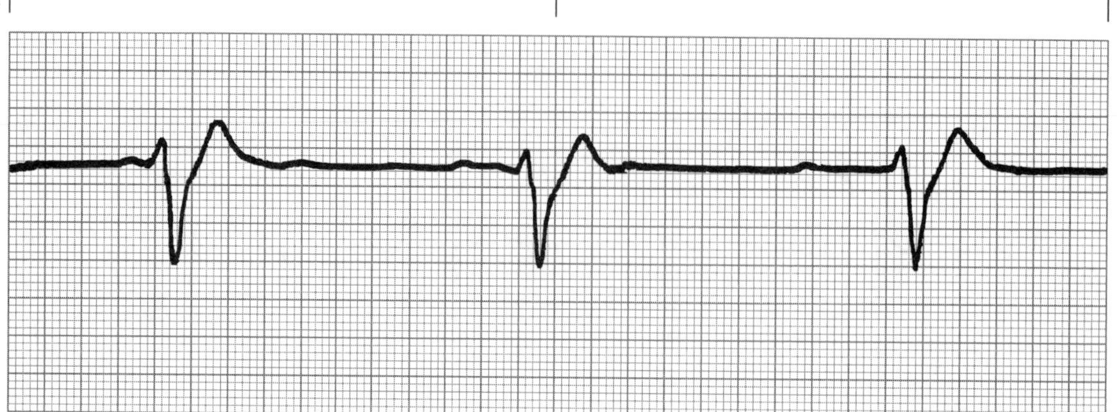

45.

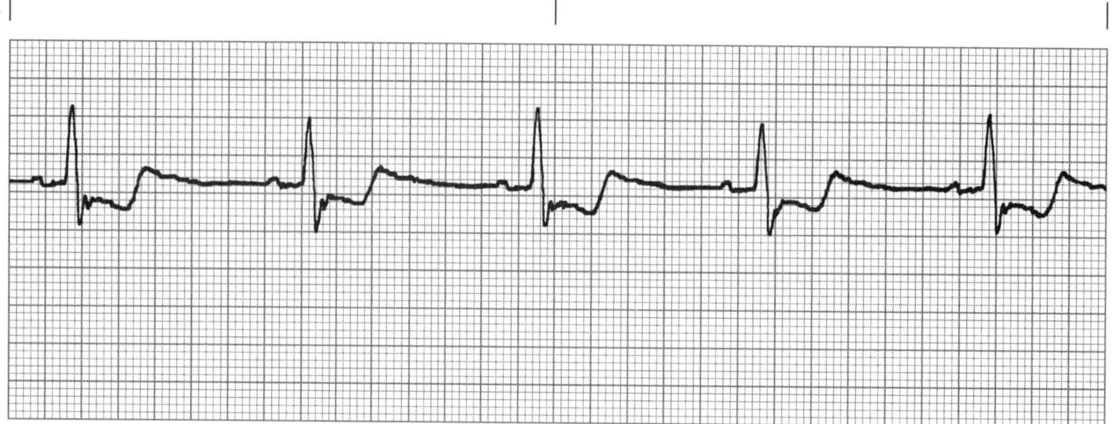

46.

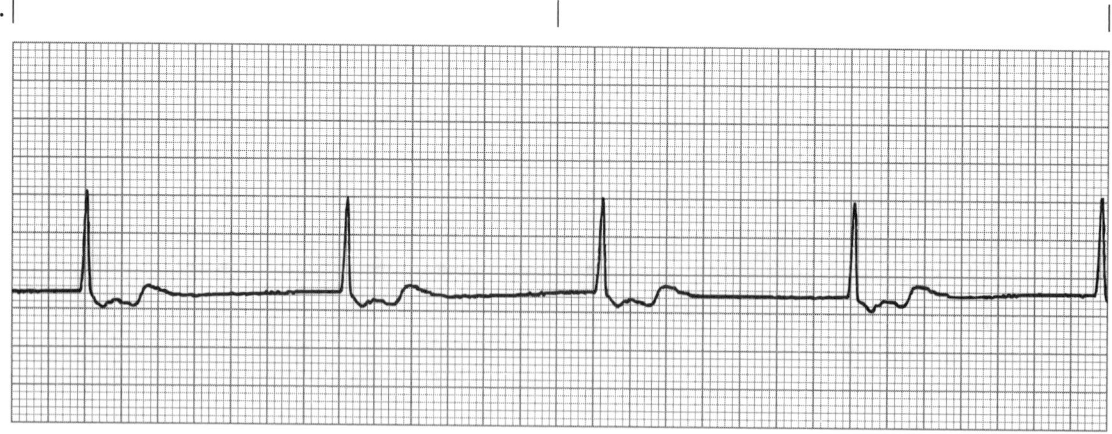

47.

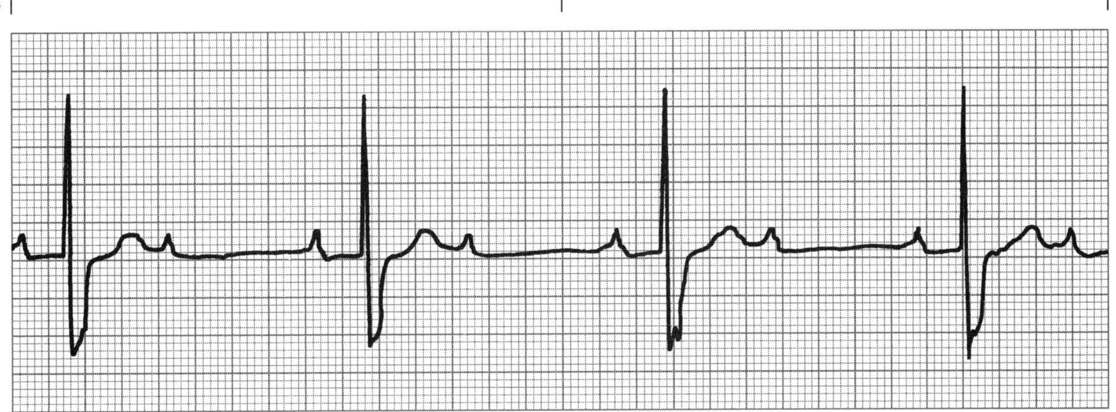

48.

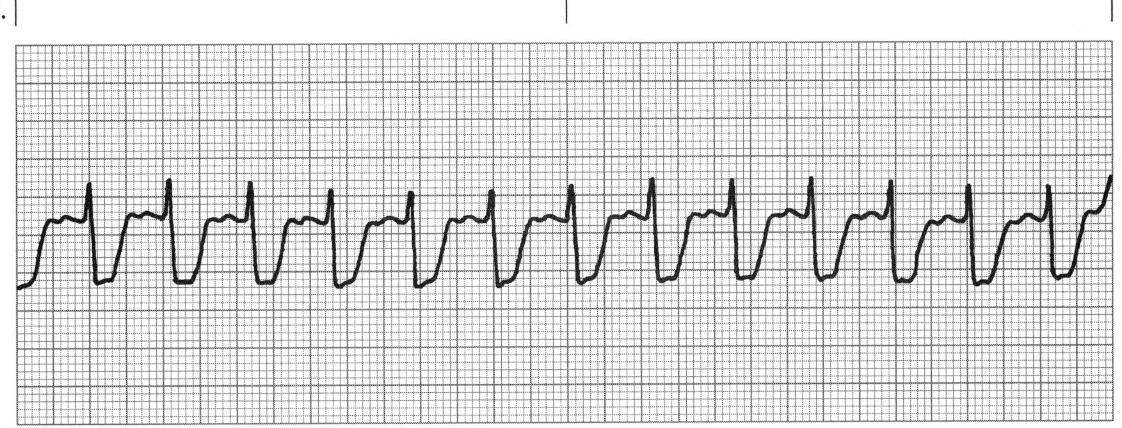

49.

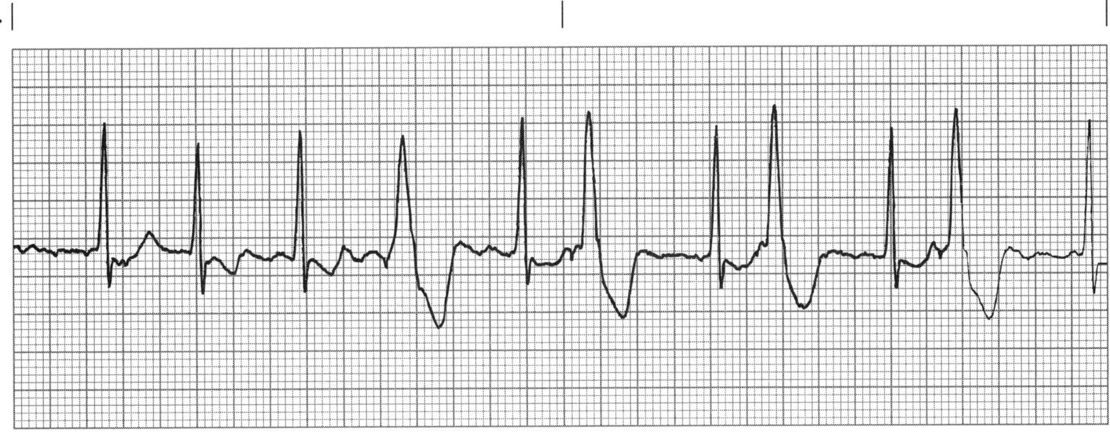

50.

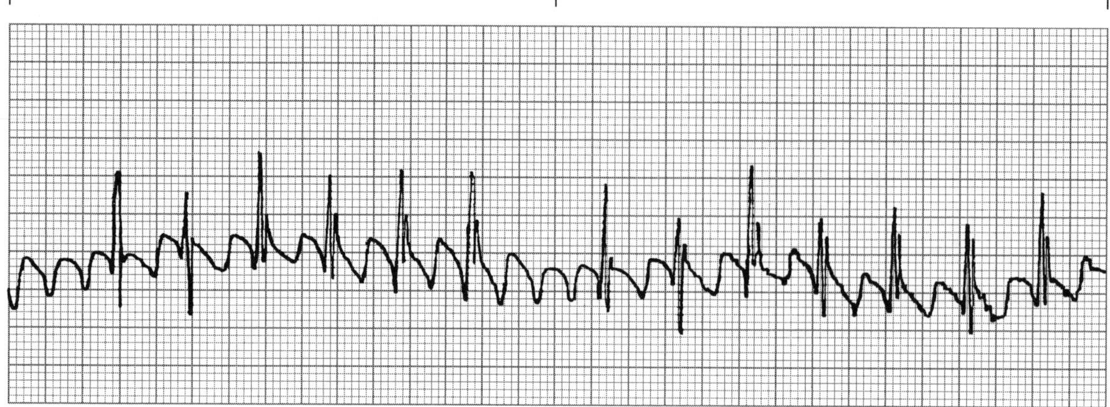

Practice Test 2 Identifying Rhythms

Name the following cardiac rhythms:

1.

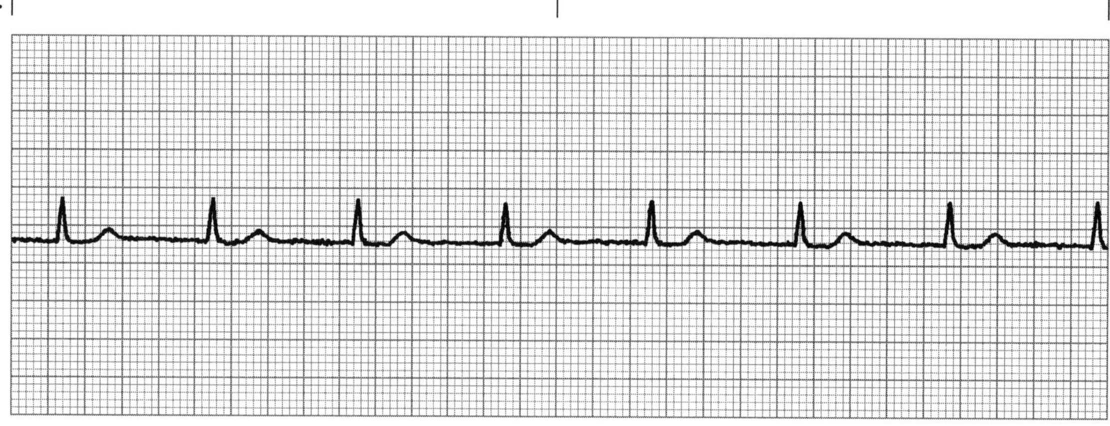

2.

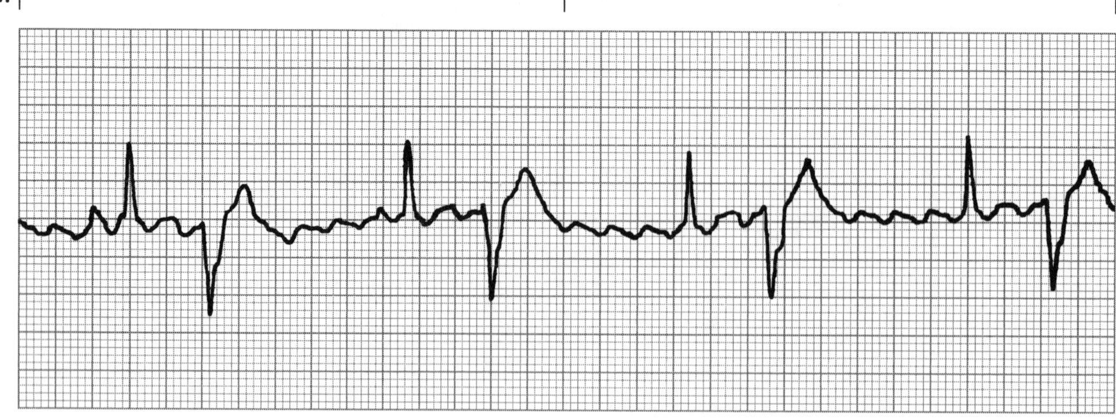

3.
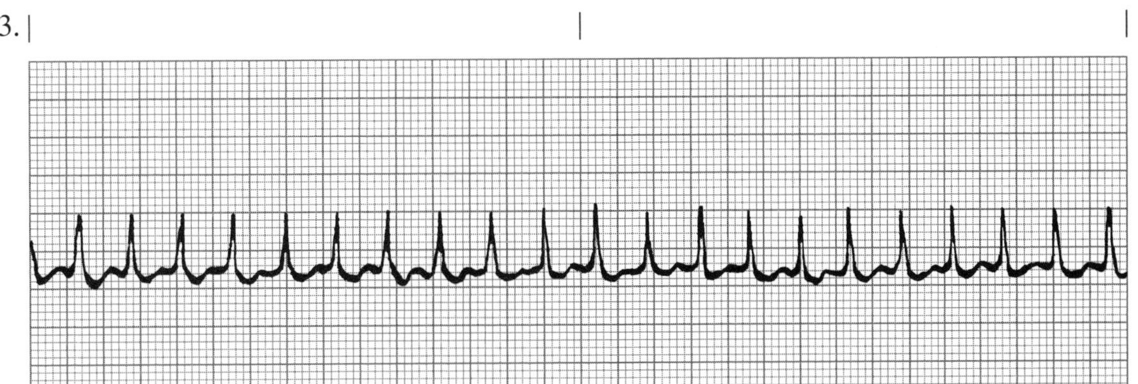

4.
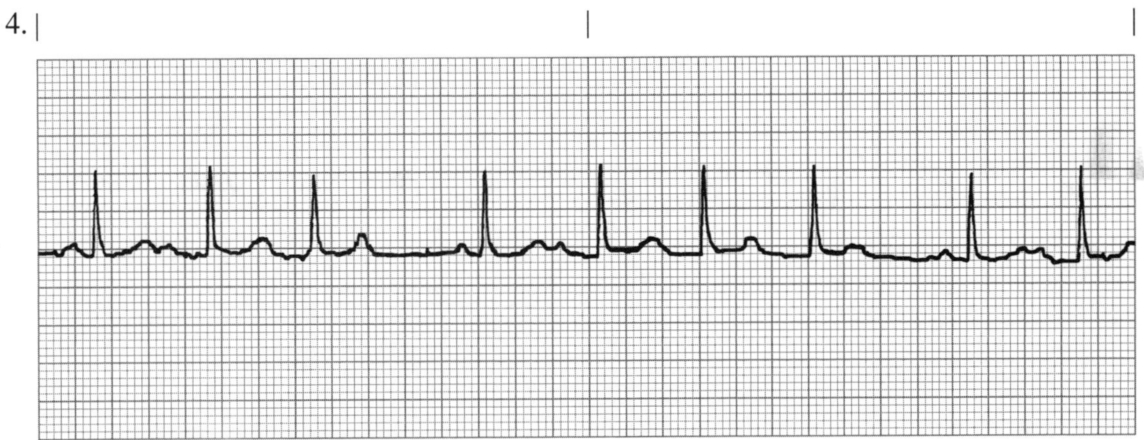

5.
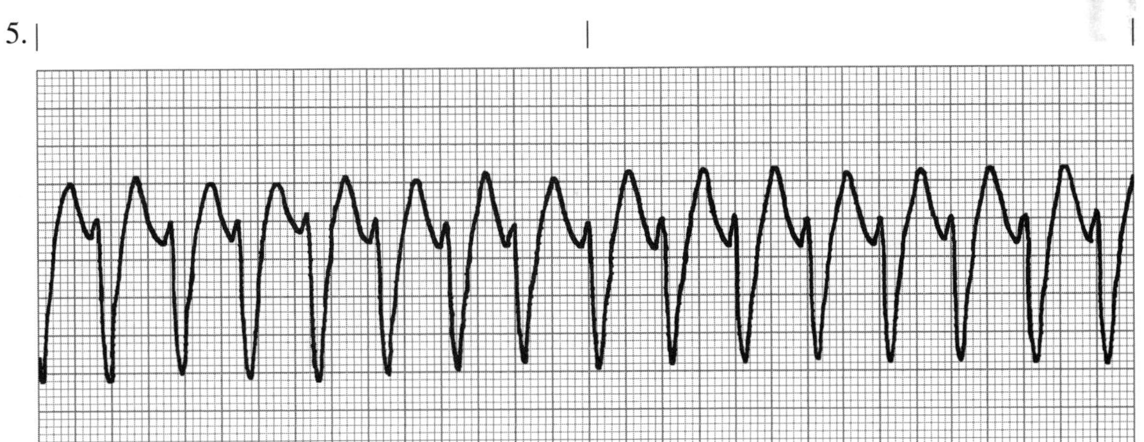

6.

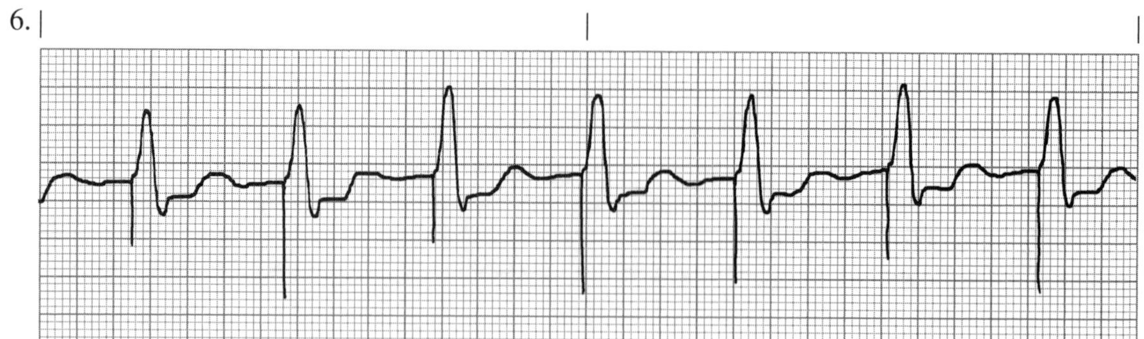

7.

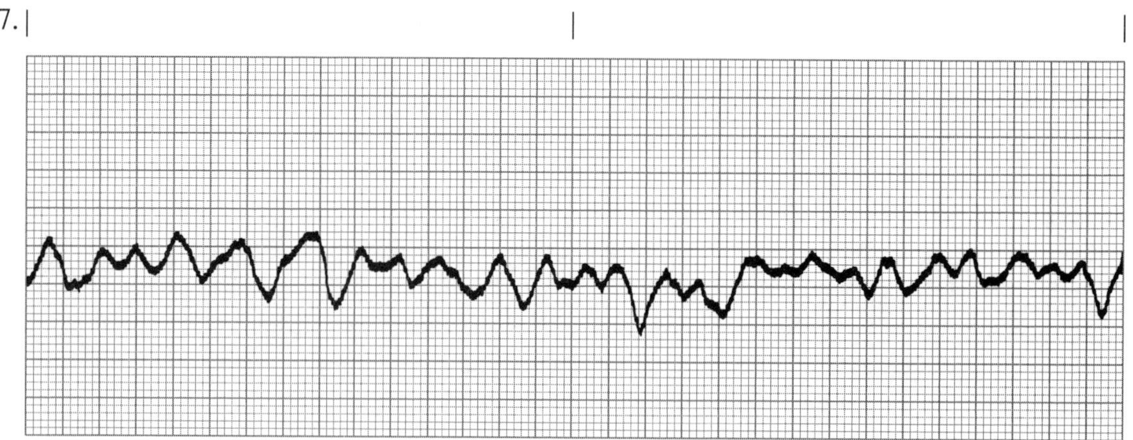

8.

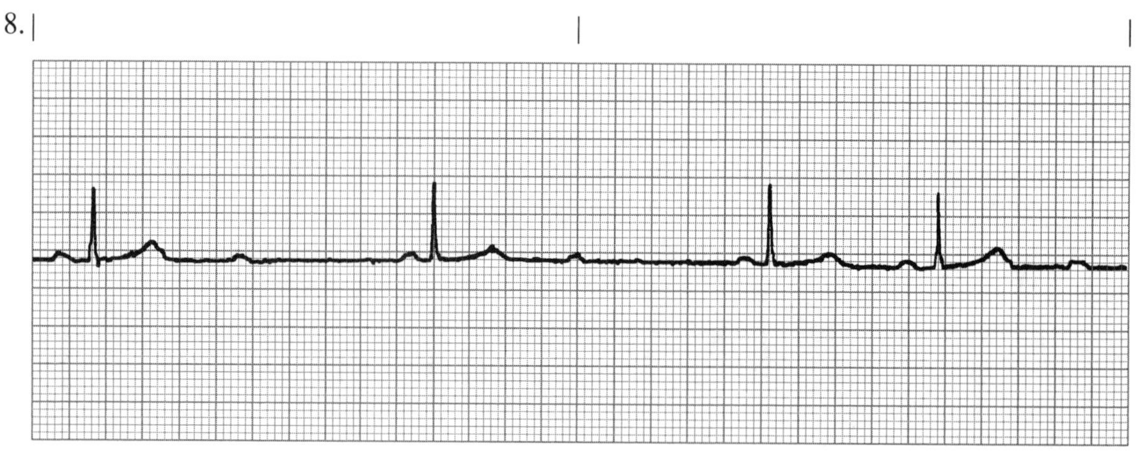

9.

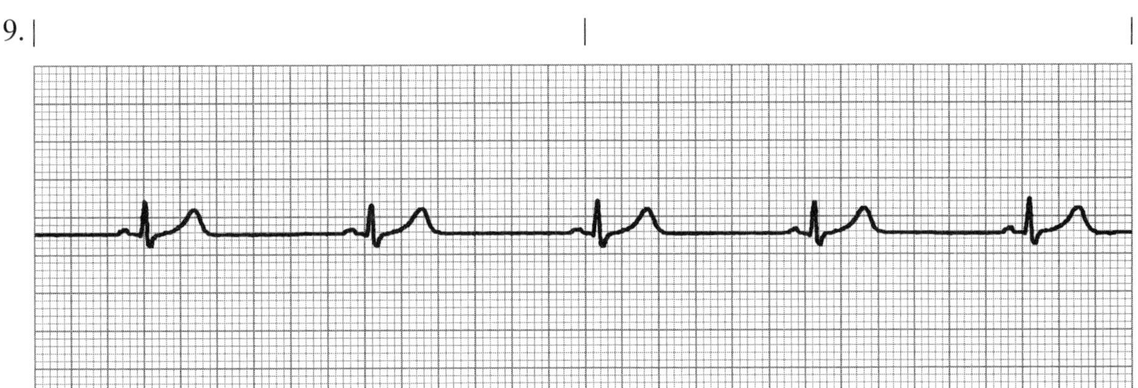

10.

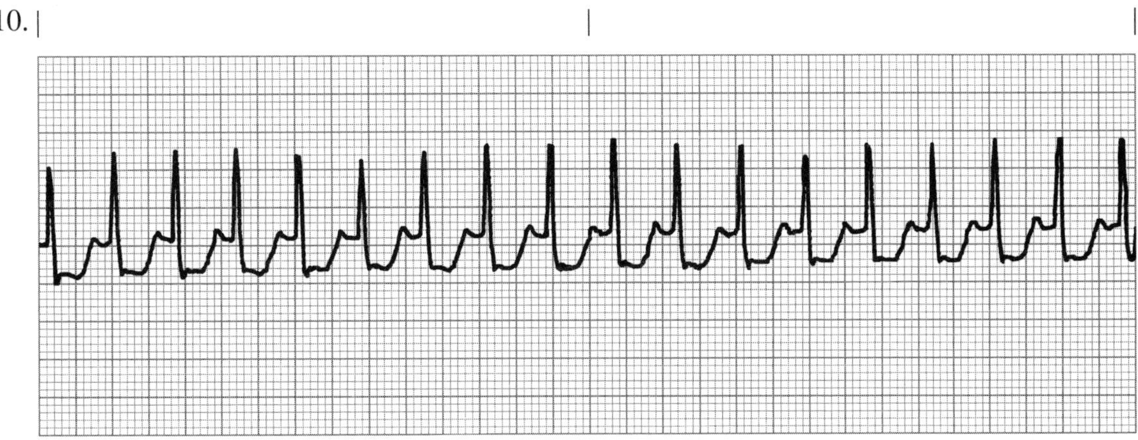

11.

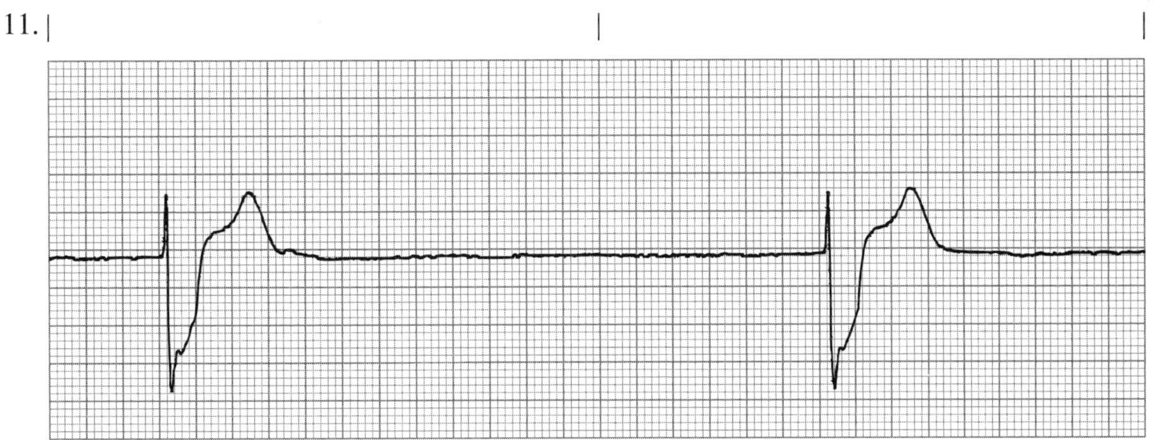

12.

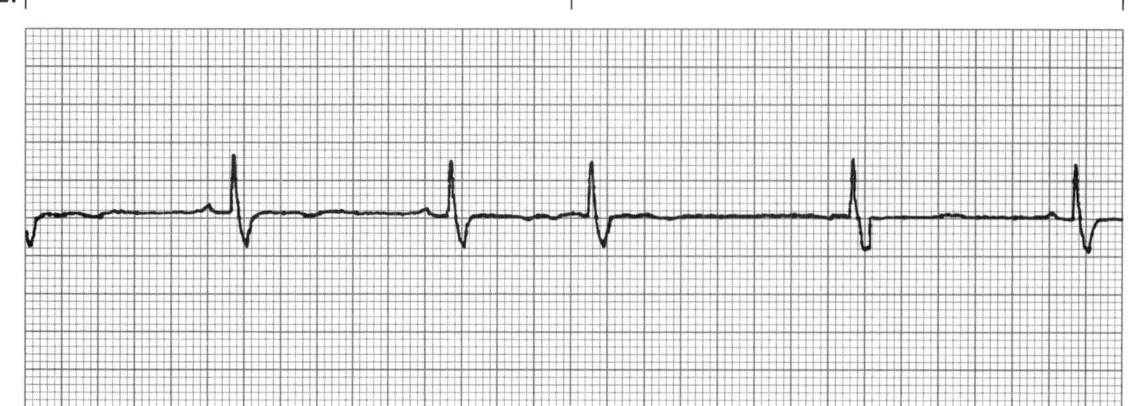

13.

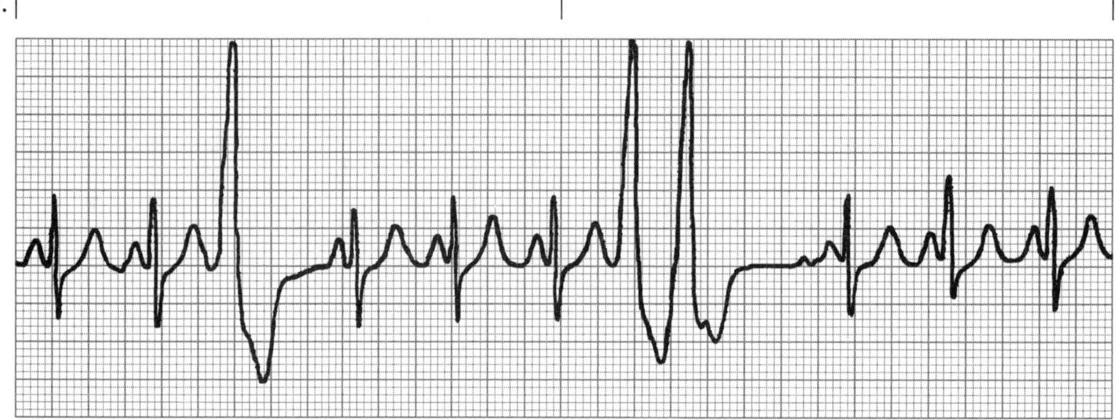

14.

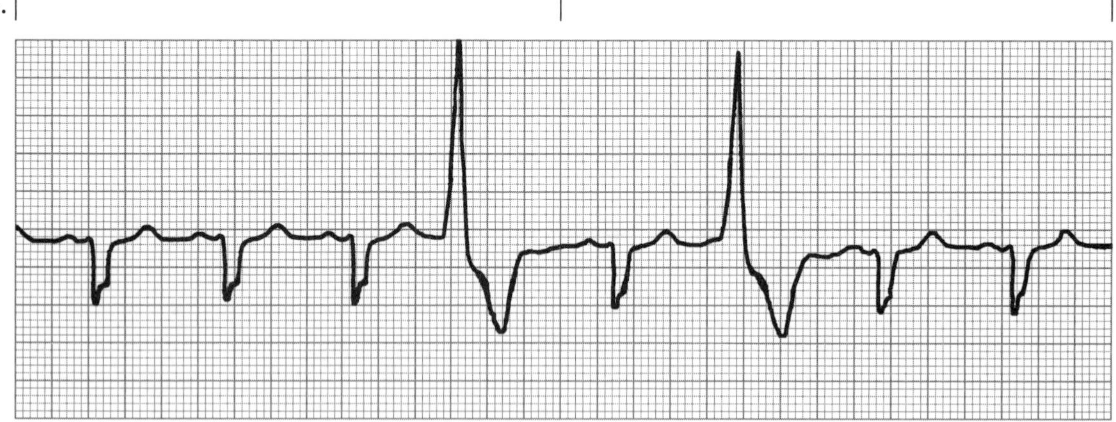

15.

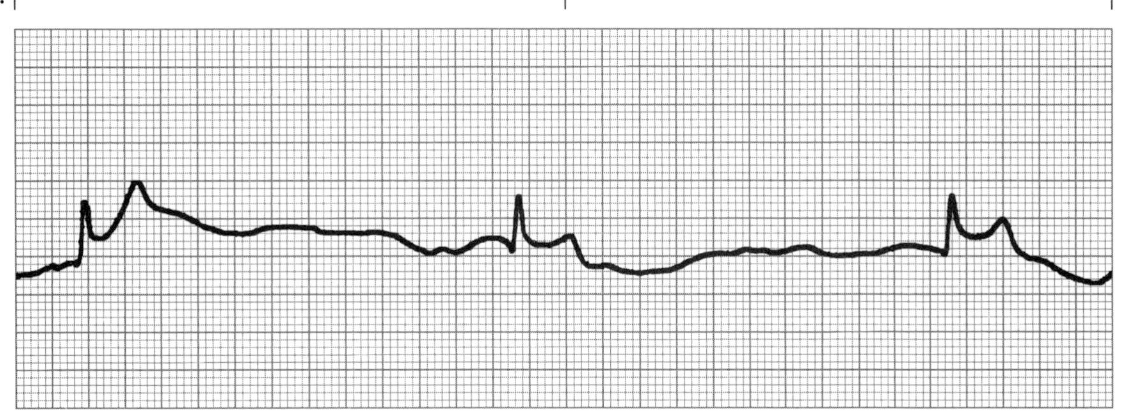

16.

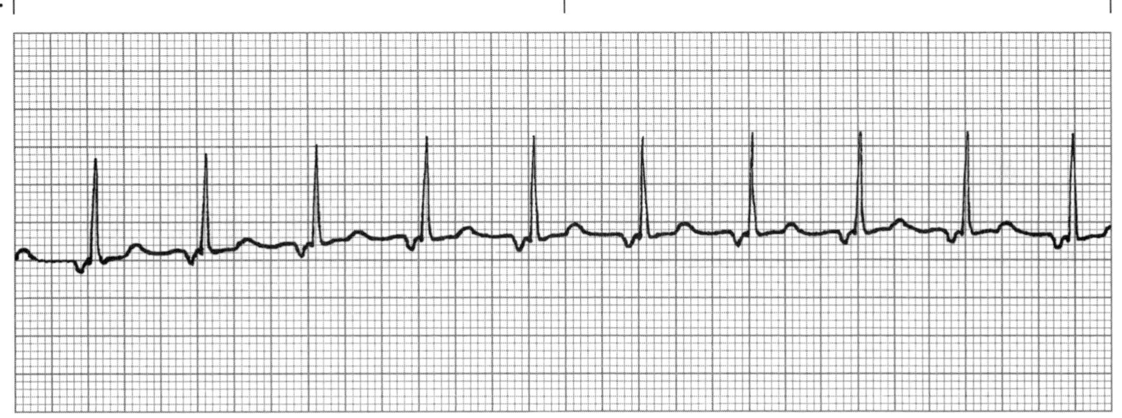

17.

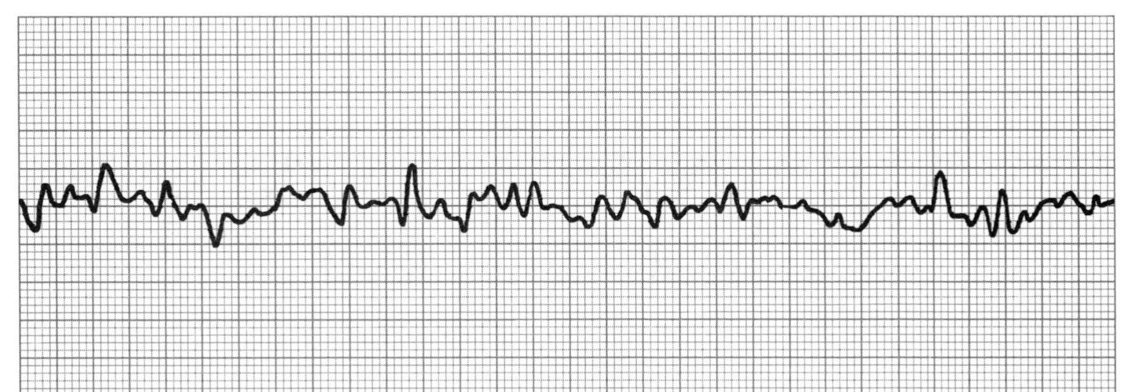

18.

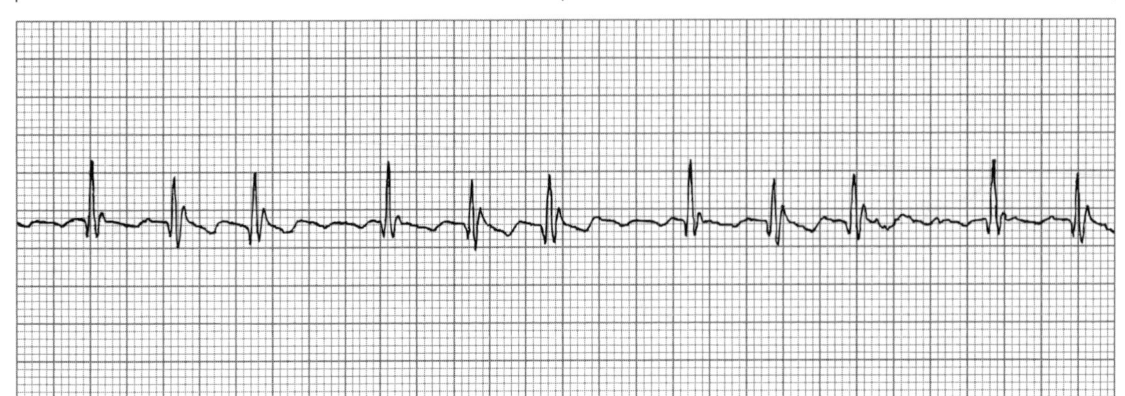

19.

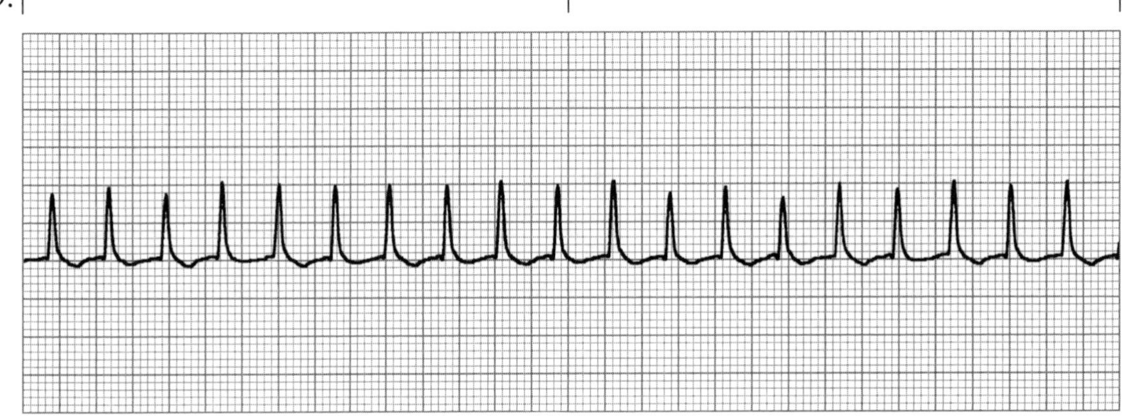

20.

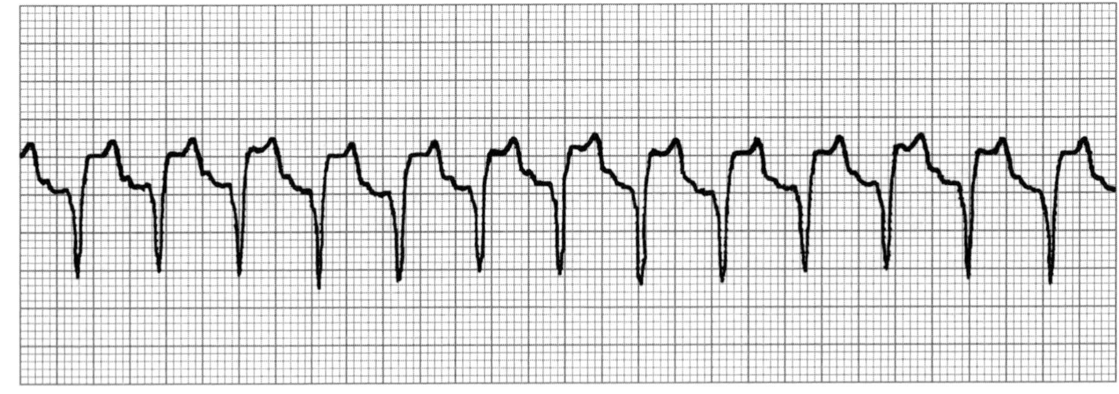

21.

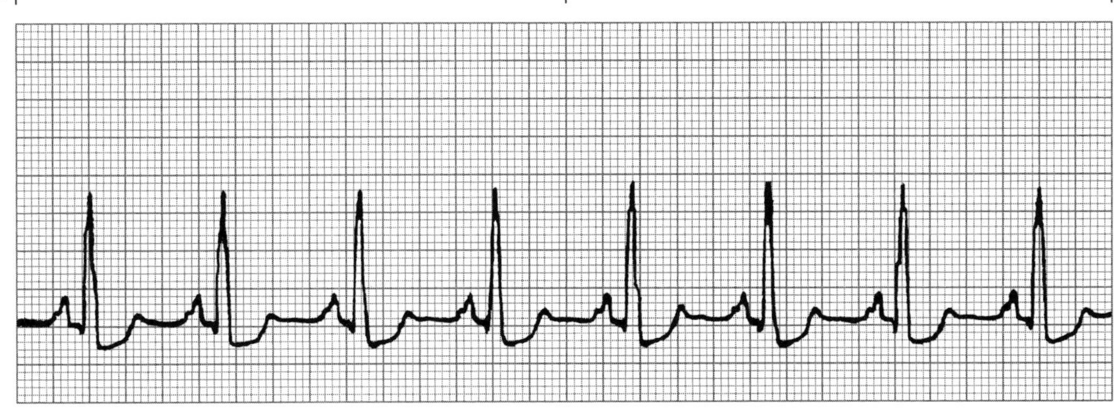

22.

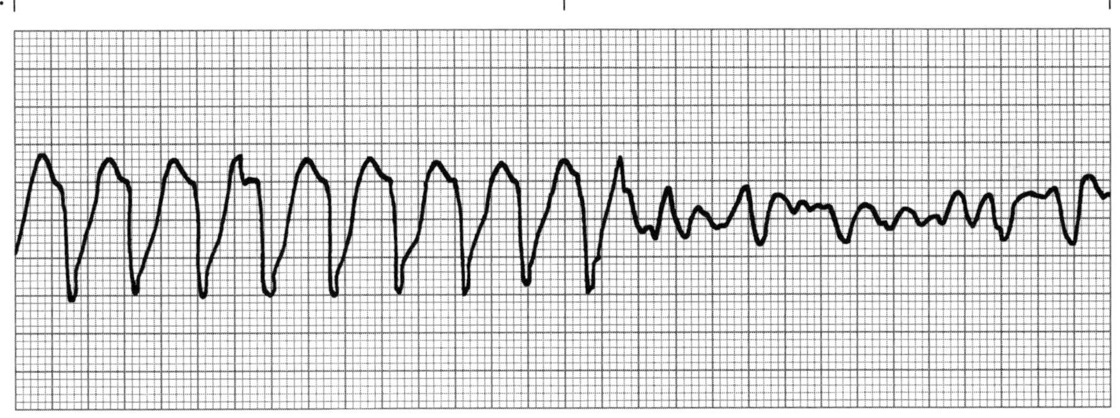

23.

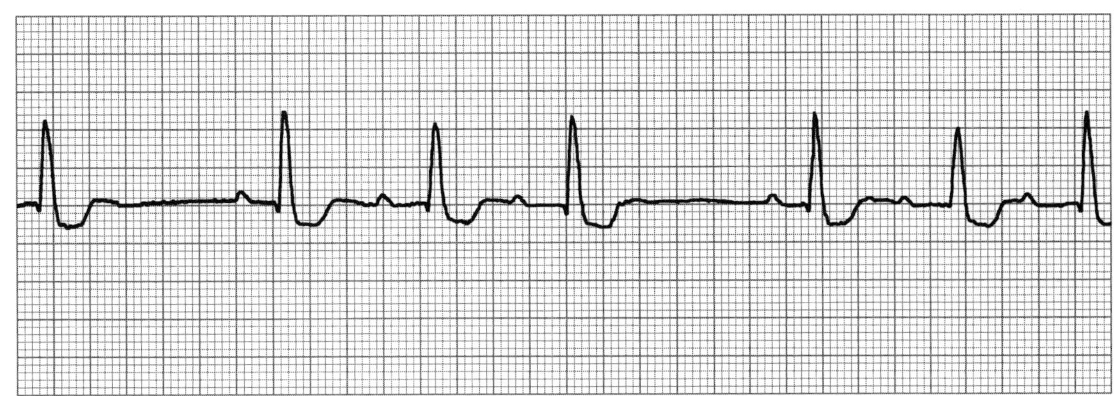

24.

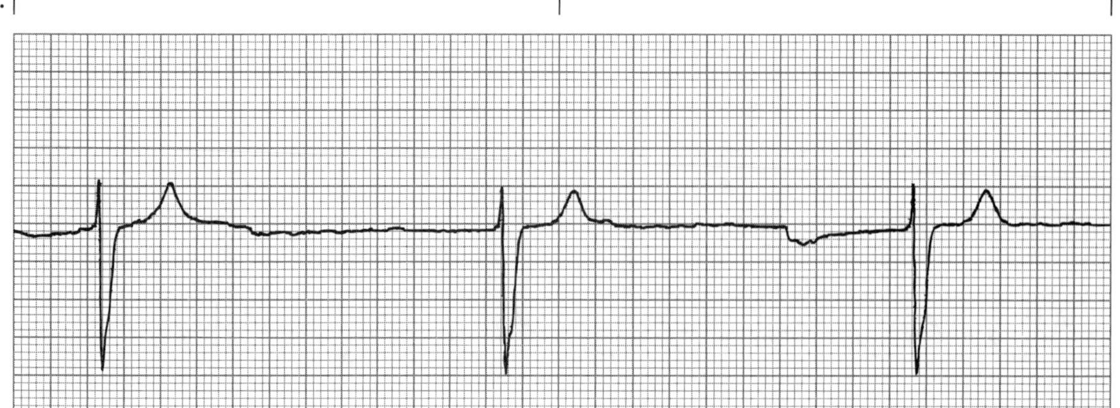

25.

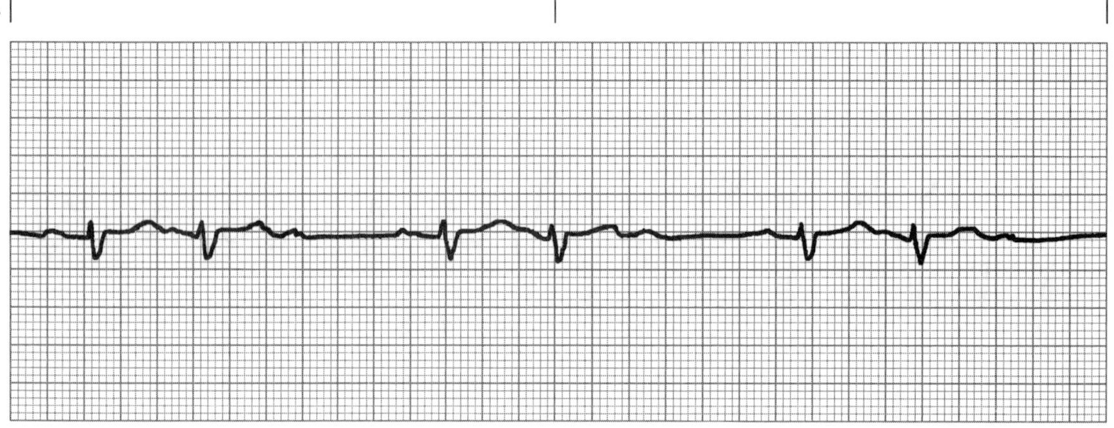

26.

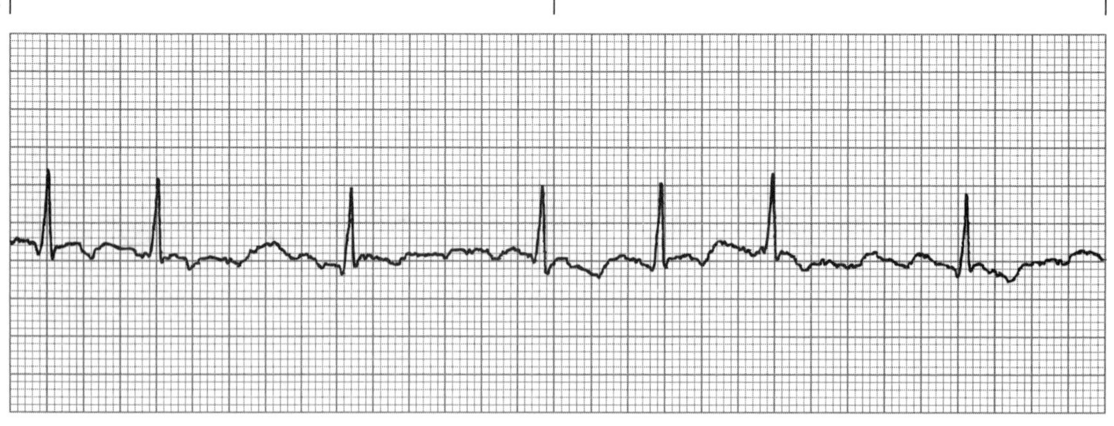

27.

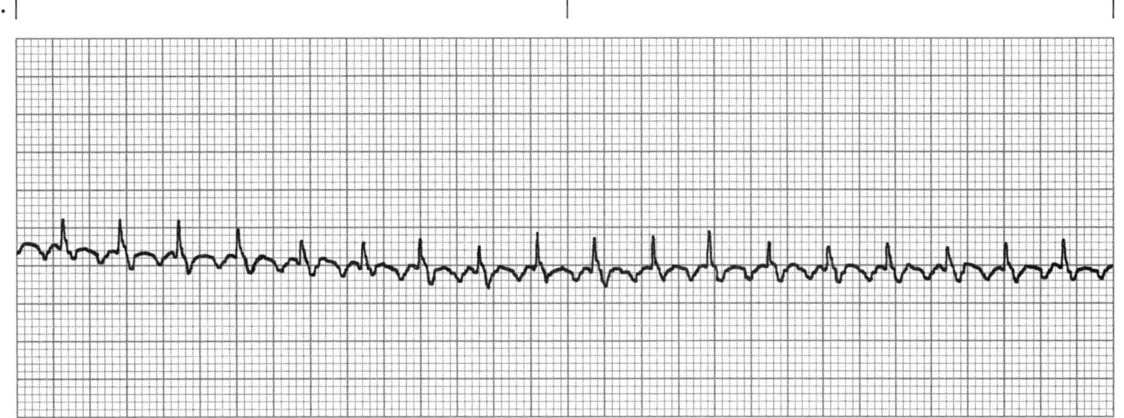

28.

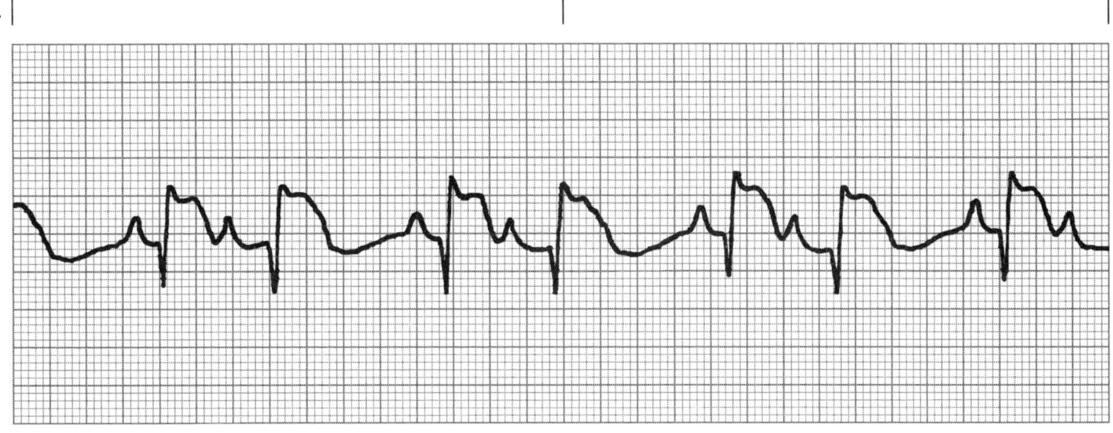

29.

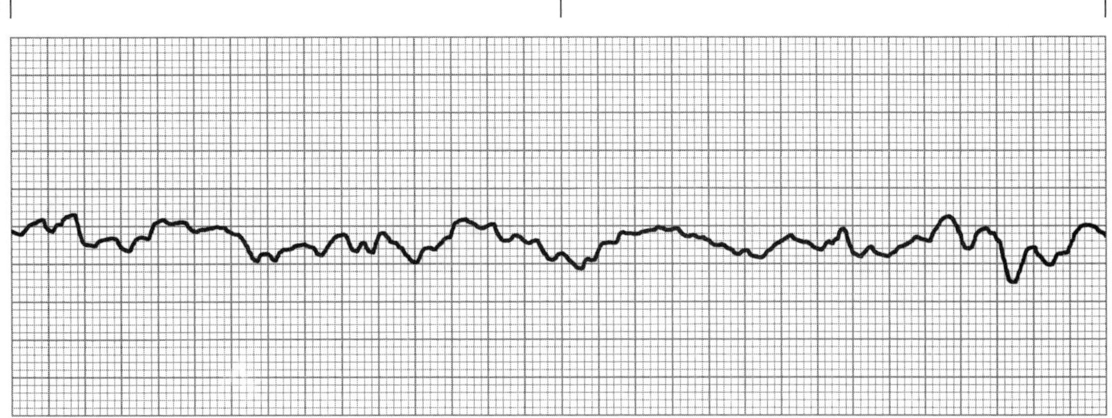

30.

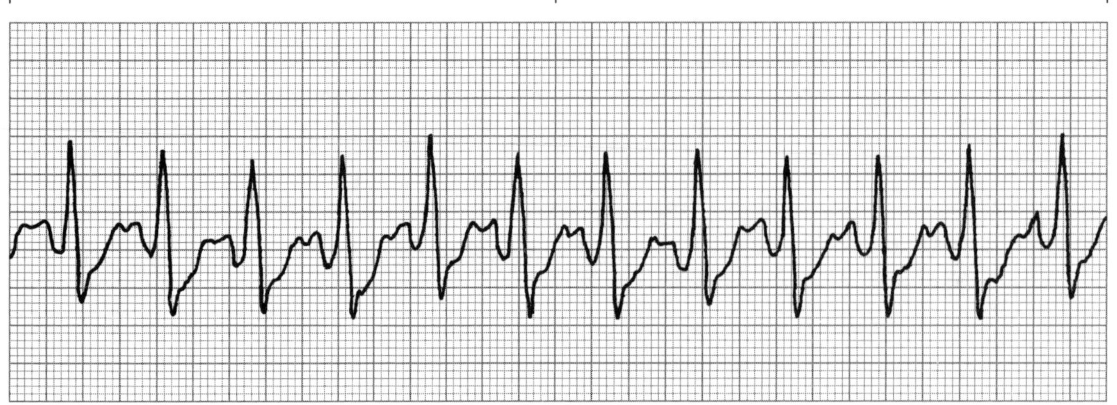

31.

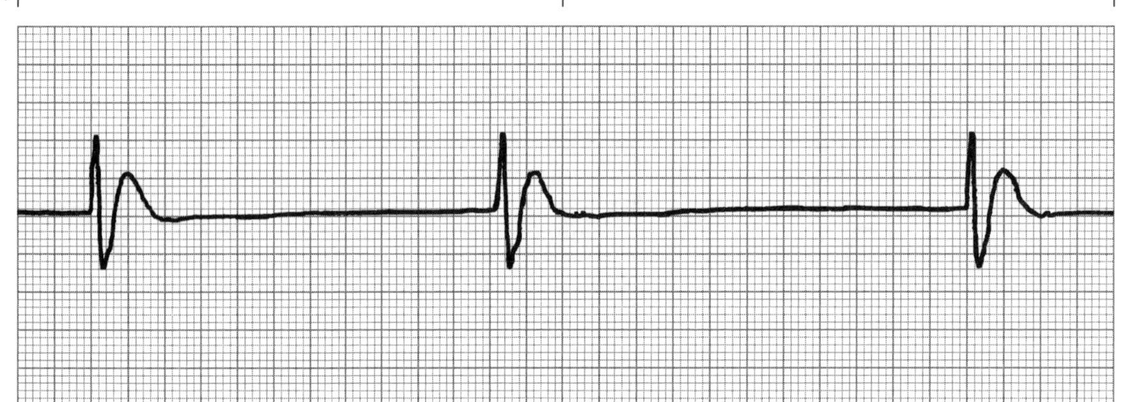

32.

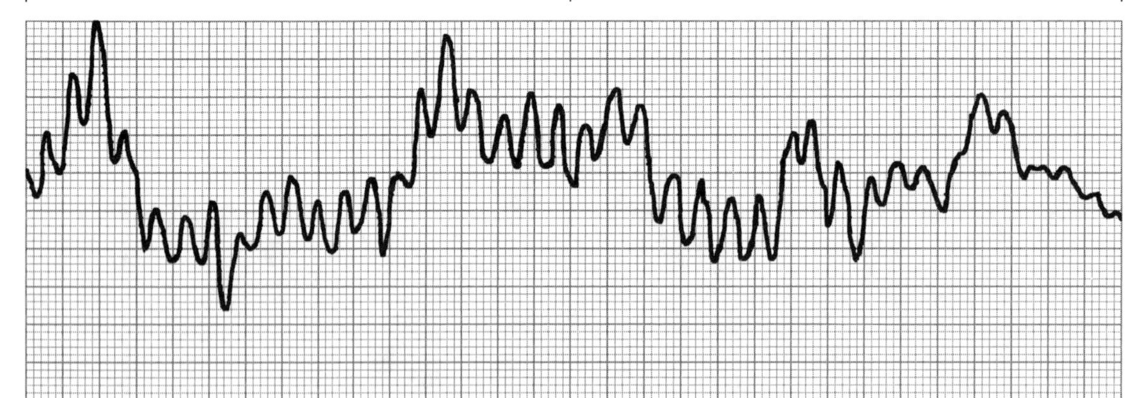

33.

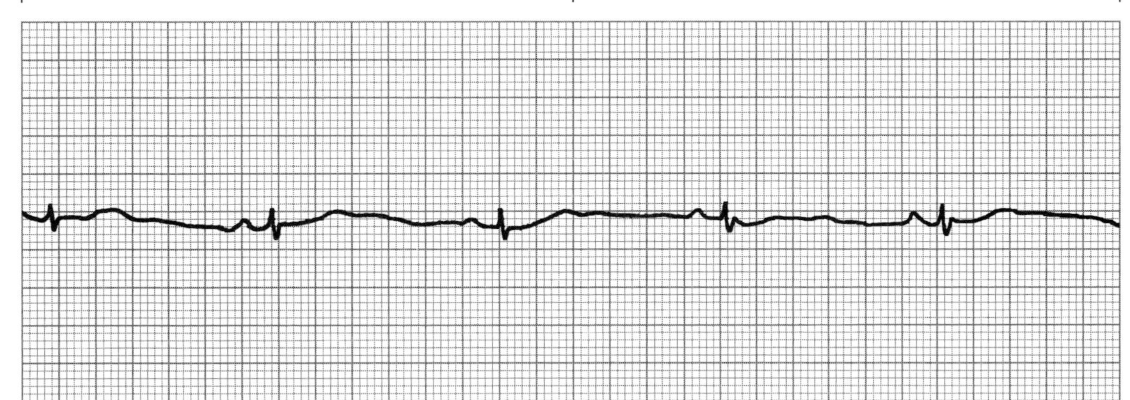

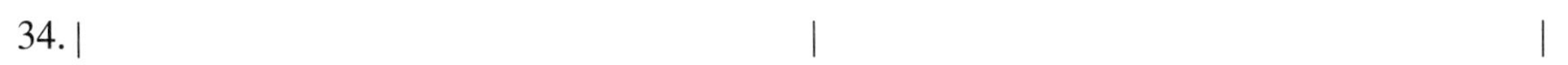
34.

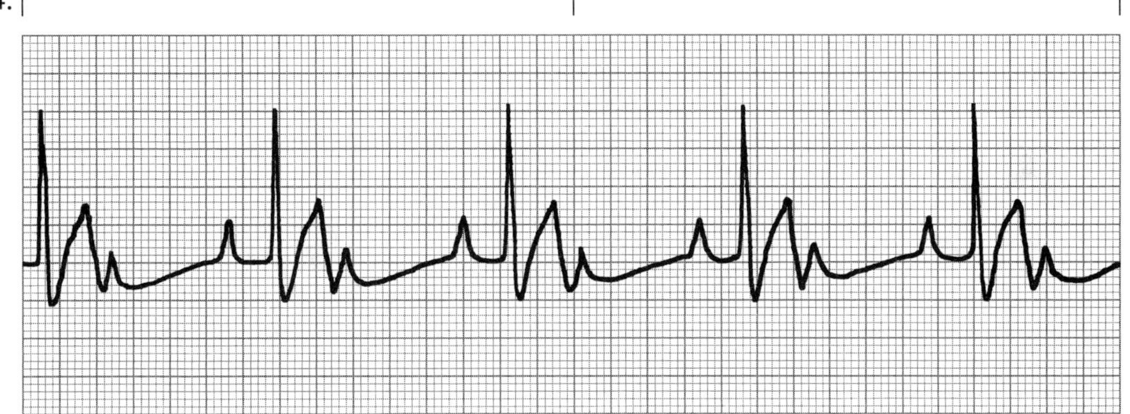

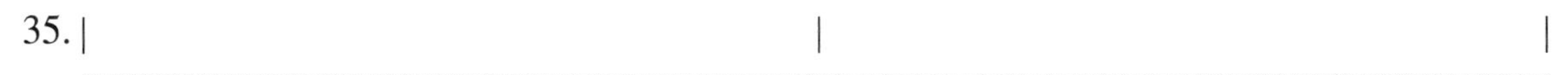
35.

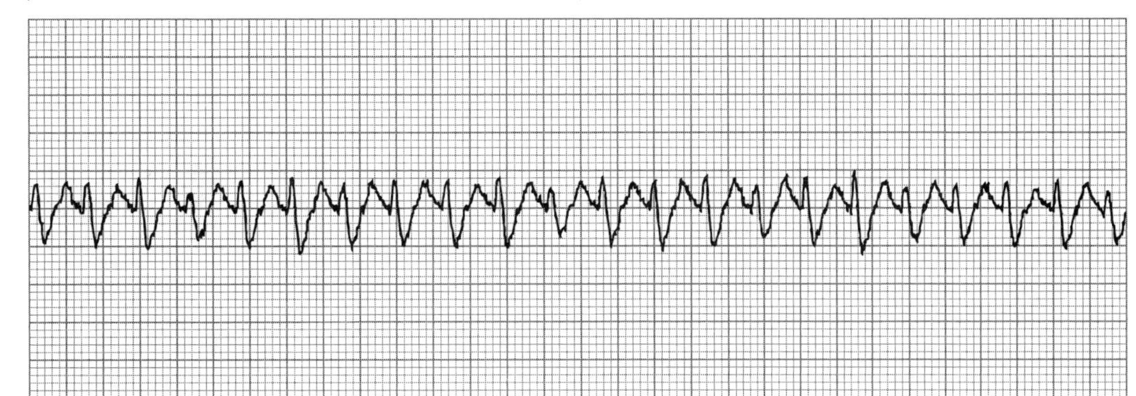

36.

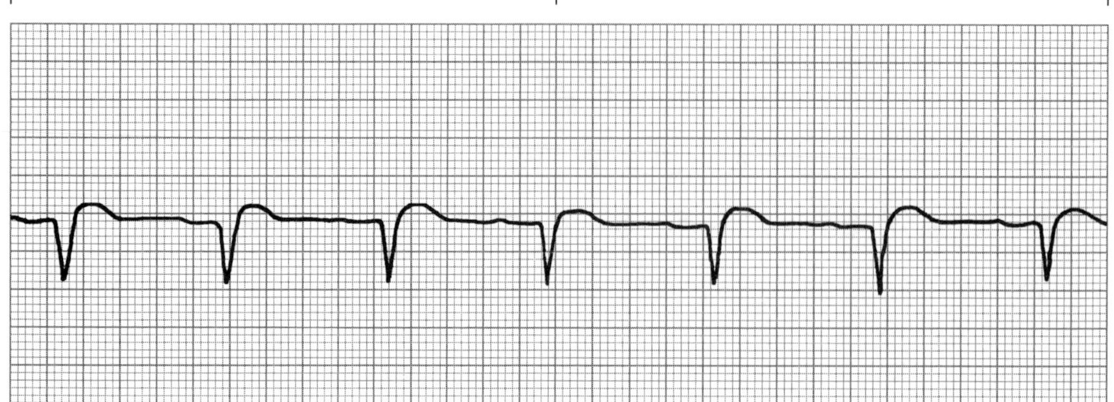

37.

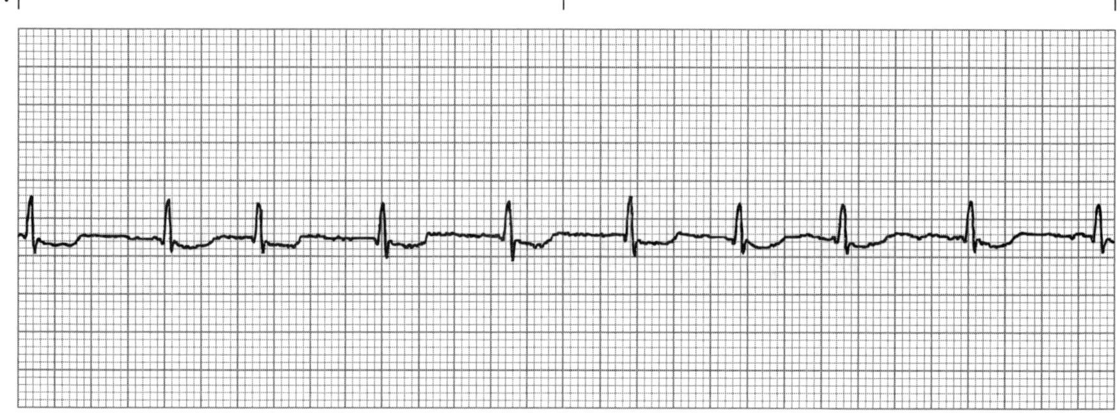

38.

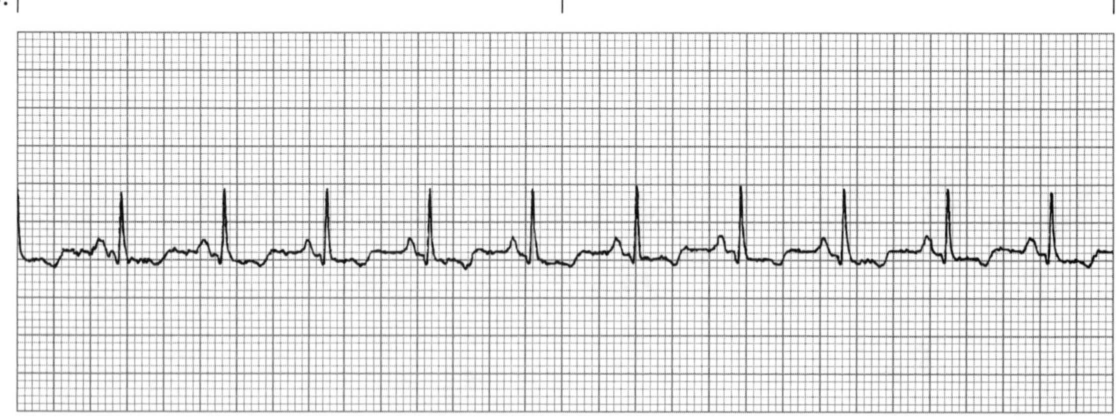

39.

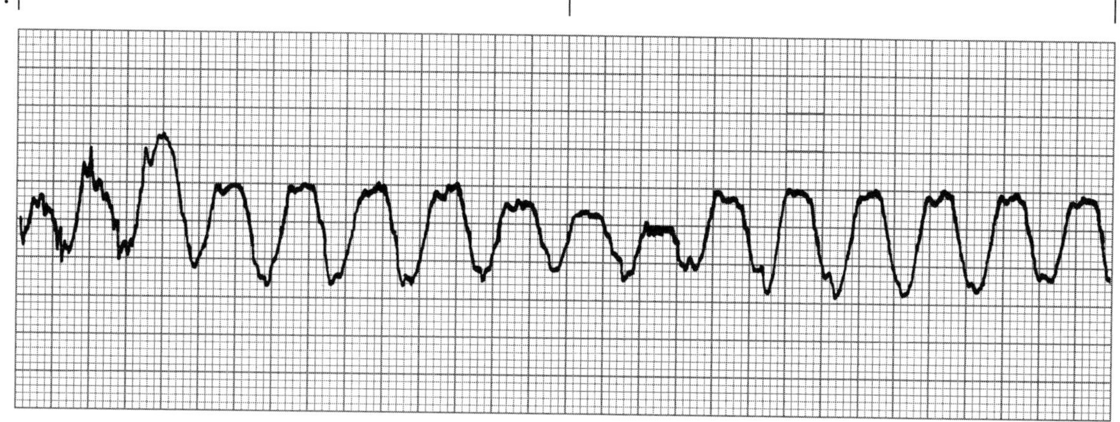

40.

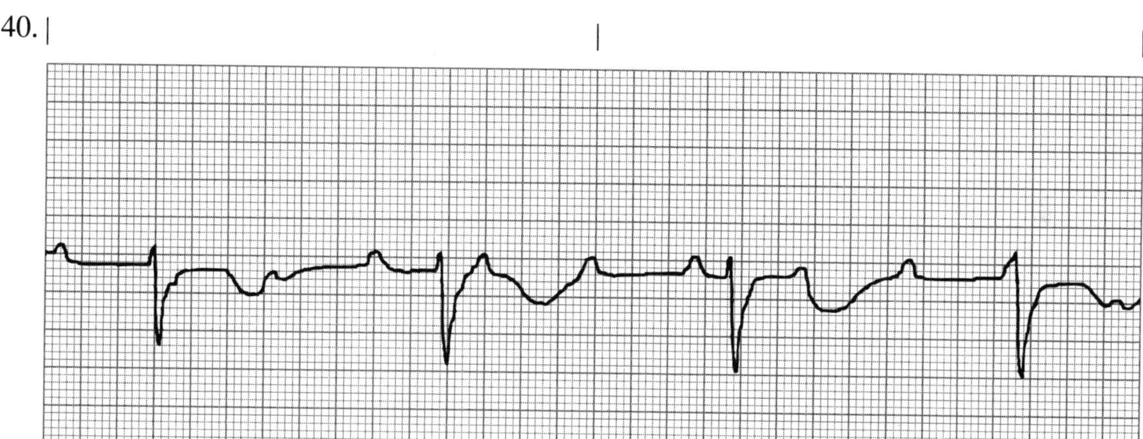

41.

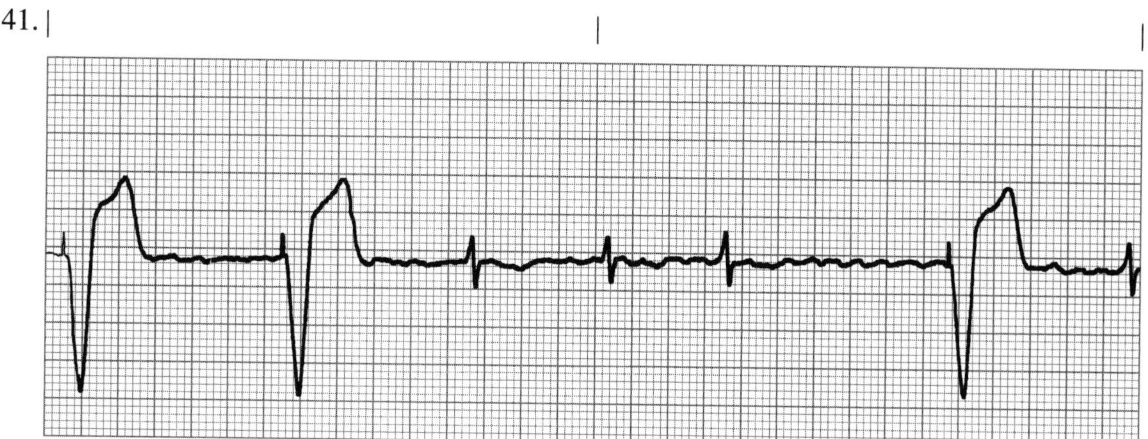

42.

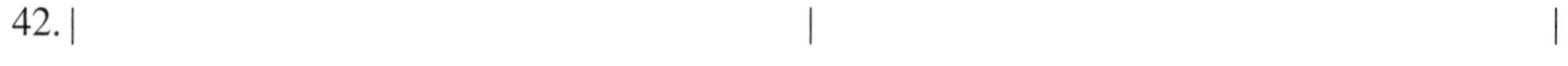

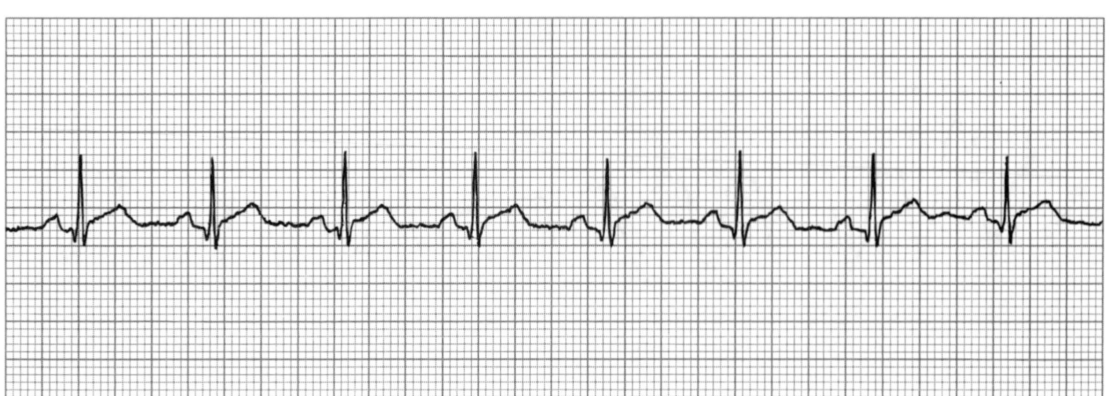

43.

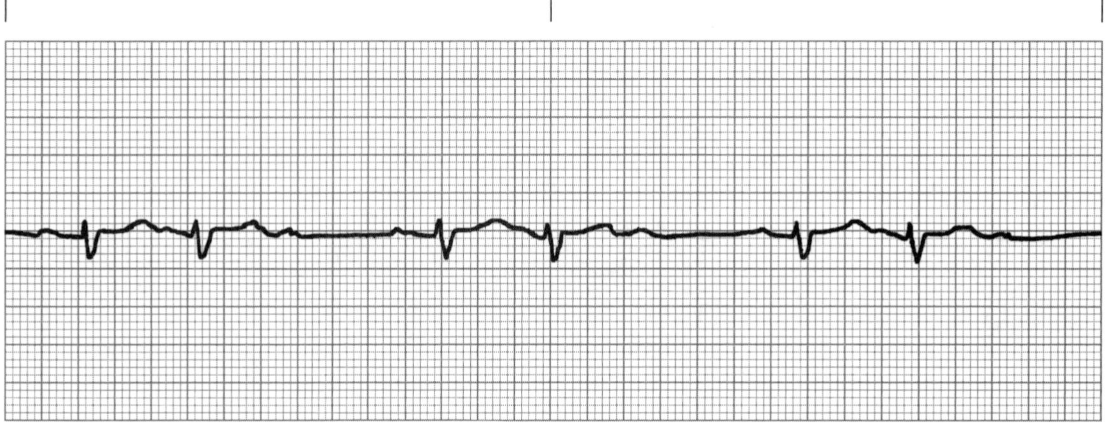

44.

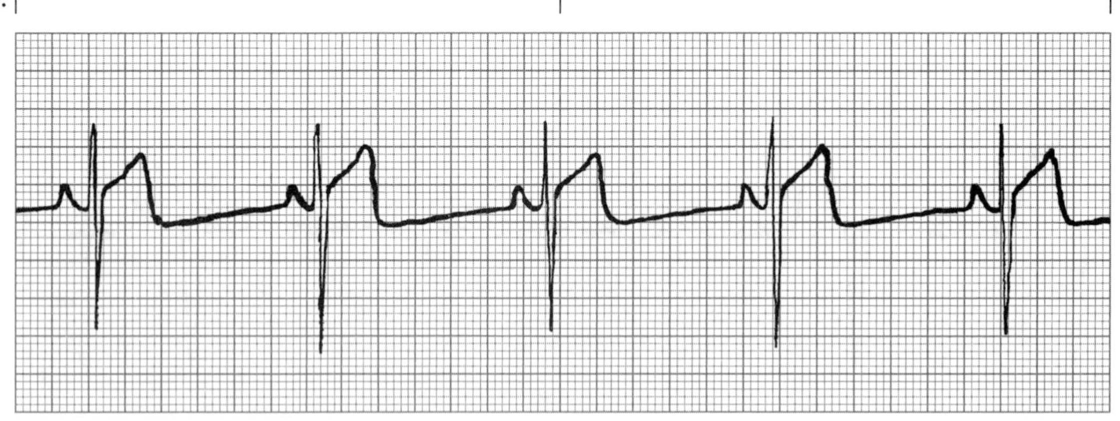

45. 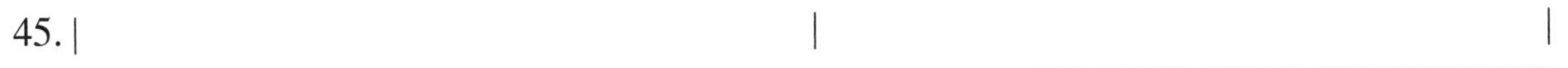

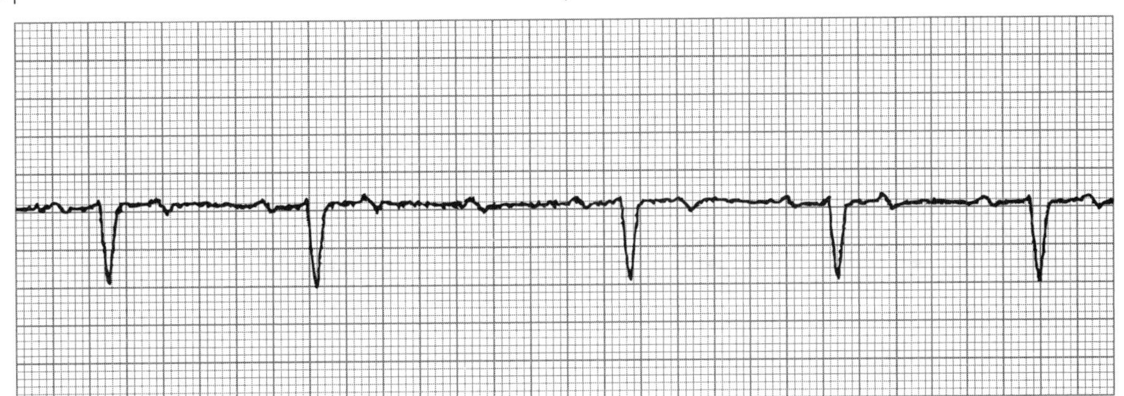

46. 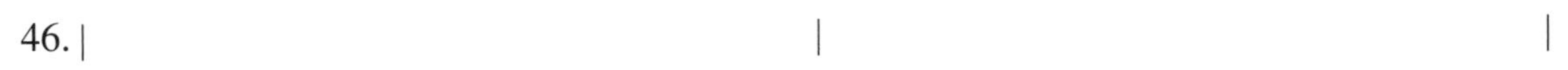

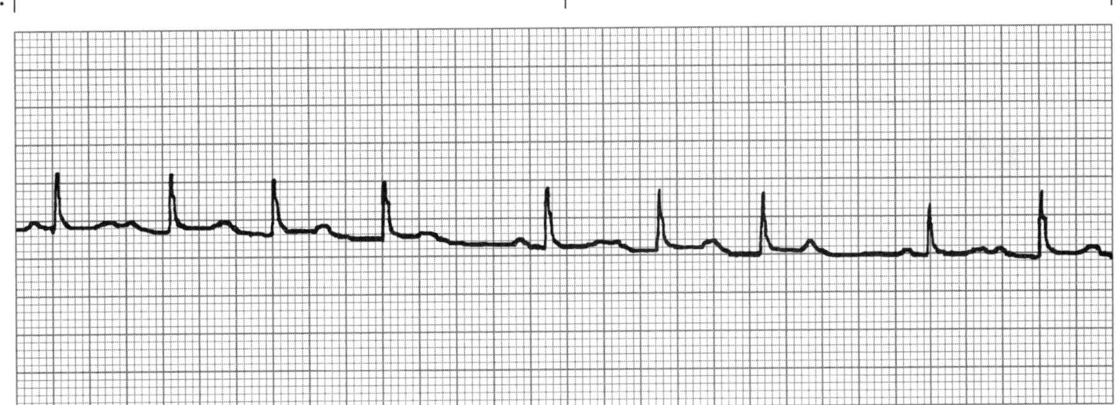

47. 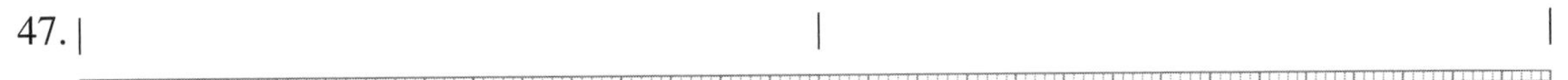

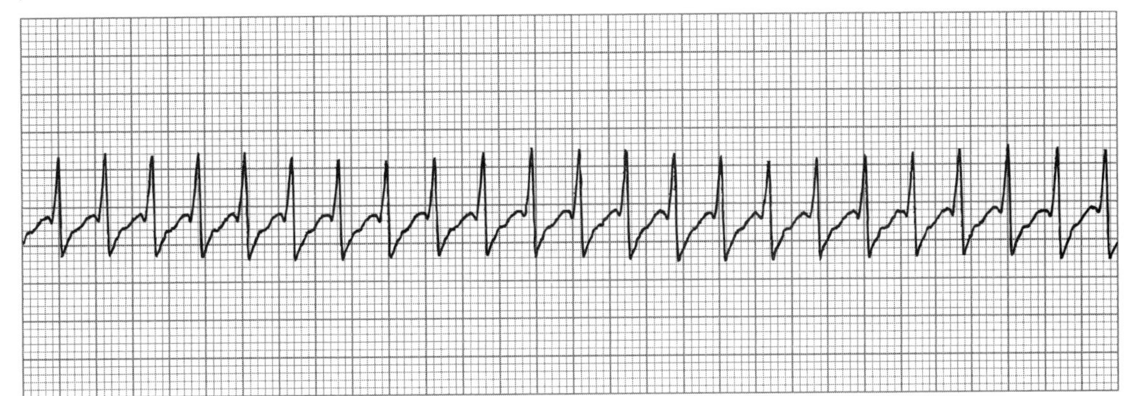

48.

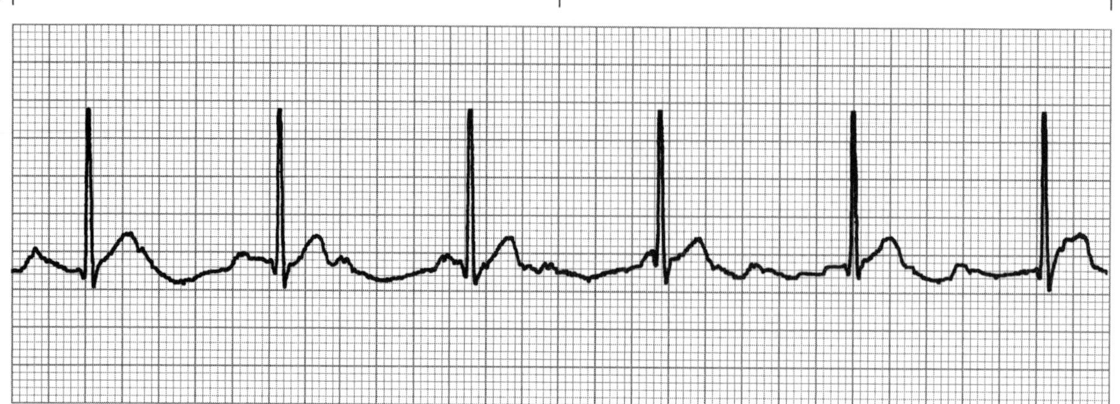

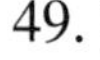

49.

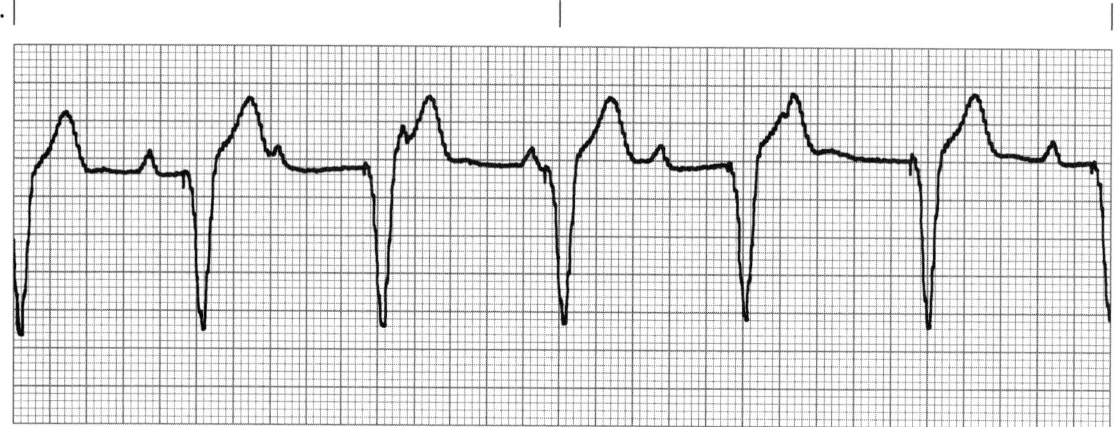

50.

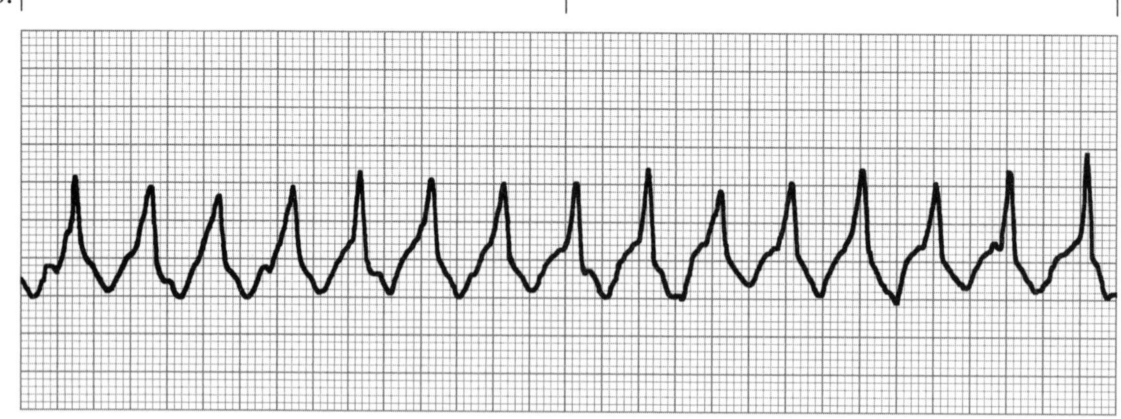

CHAPTER 4

12-Lead ECGs

12-Lead ECGs as a Diagnostic Tool

In the United States the terms EKG and ECG are interchangeable. This section is designed to be a very basic overview of understanding the 12-lead ECG. Fully understanding and interpreting the 12-lead ECG requires more hours of training than the entire ACLS course. Thus, definitive interpretation should be accomplished by an experienced skilled clinician. The goal of this section is to have the bedside clinician recognize three events, which require further investigation: myocardial ischemia (seen in angina or early AMI), myocardial injury (seen in active AMIs), and infarction (seen as a specific section of myocardial muscle dies). While some ACLS courses may only mention AMI, the clinician should be somewhat familiar with the other conditions.

ECG interpretation still begins with evaluating the limb leads or "rhythm strips" to determine the origin of the rhythm (sinus, atrial, junctional, or ventricular) rate and regularity. Although sometimes addressed in combination, stabilizing the patient's rate and rhythm generally takes precedence over managing 12-lead ECG complications. The standard is that the rhythm should be monitored immediately during the initial assessment and the 12-lead accomplished within the first 10 minutes.

The 12-lead ECG utilizes 10 electrode wires to take a brief snapshot of each specific area of the heart with an emphasis on the left ventricle, the origin of most myocardial infarction. Upon printing to paper, the clinician is given a 2½-second view from each lead (about three complexes). By understanding a bit about anatomy and lead placement the clinician is able to determine if there is ischemia, injury, or infarction occurring to specific regions of the myocardium by simply evaluating the ST segment. Though 12-lead ECGs are quite effective, it should be emphasized this is merely one tool in the arsenal of managing patients. Treatment is based on the patient's symptoms, presentation, history, and other clinical findings. Remember, treat the patient, not just the machine.

LEAD PLACEMENT

Along with limb leads—Right Arm (white), Left Arm (black), Right Leg (green), and Left Leg (red), the precordial or V-leads are placed as shown in Figure 4-1.

THE 12-LEAD PRINTOUT

On the 12-lead printout the complexes may look the same or significantly different than the standard 3-lead complexes for the same patient. This is due to the fact that each "lead" (wire) takes a quick snapshot of the myocardium from its

Figure 4-1 Note that the V4 or V5 lead can be moved to the right side to evaluate that area if needed

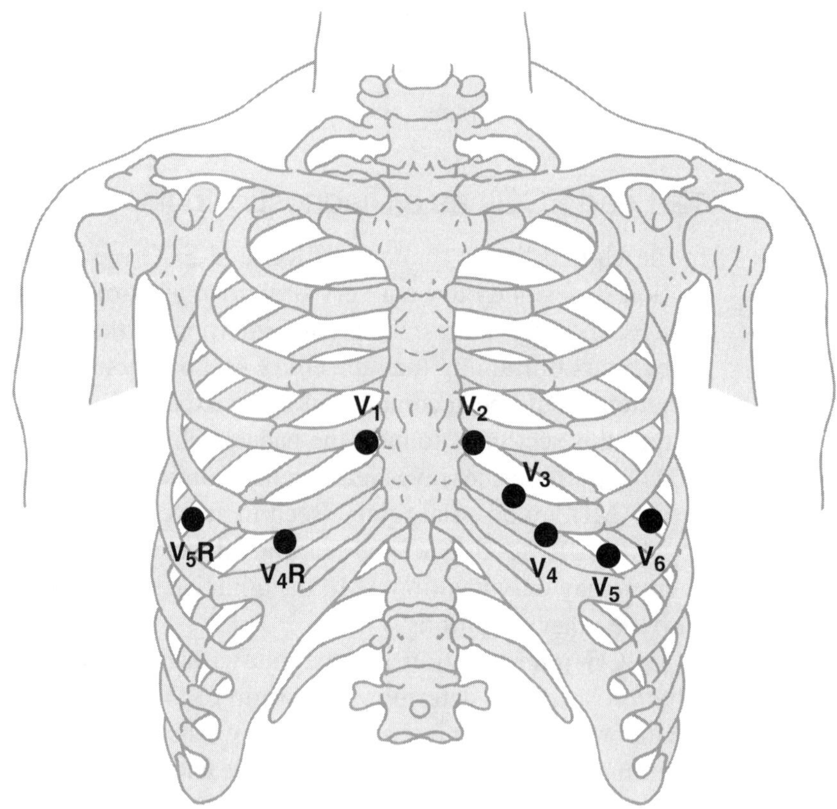

V_1—4th intercostal space, right of the sternum
V_2—4th intercostal space, left of the sternum
V_3—5th intercostal space, halfway between V_2 and V_4
V_4—5th intercostal space, left midclavicular line
V_5—5th intercostal space, left anterior axillary line
V_6—5th intercostal space, left midaxillary line
V_4R—5th intercostal space, right midclavicular line
V_5R—5th intercostal space, right anterior axillary line

unique angle in relation to the heart with an emphasis on the left ventricle. Also, the "filtering system" on a 12-lead monitor is more complex than a 3-lead rhythm strip.

By simply looking at the location of the precordial or V-leads in relation to where the heart is located in the chest it is easy to localize which area each lead views:

V1 or V2 view the septal wall

V3 and V4 view the anterior wall of the left ventricle

V5 and V6 view the lateral wall of the left ventricle

The limb leads and what is called the augmented voltage (aVR, aVF, aVL) look either from the limbs through the heart (standard lead I, II, III) or from the heart towards the limbs; the ECG machine must "augment" the power in order to do this, thus the terms: aVR (augmented voltage right), aVL (augmented voltage left), aVF (augmented voltage foot).

The specific leads are viewed in the following manner:

Lead II, III, aVF View the inferior wall of the left ventricle. Due to the anatomical location of the heart these leads can also view the right ventricle; thus an AMI showing in these leads may require the V4 or V5 lead be moved to the same spot on the right side of the chest, and an additional ECG be run to evaluate the right ventricle as well. These patients may become seriously hypotensive if nitroglycerine is administered.

Lead I, aVL View the lateral wall of the left ventricle.

Quick Tip

The acronym **SALI** can be used to remember the location each group of leads is able to view:

S Septal wall V1, V2.

A Anterior left ventricle V3, V4.

L Lateral left ventricle V5, V6; also I and aVL.

I Inferior left ventricle II, III, and aVF.

Note the standard 12-lead printout and location of each lead view (Figure 4-2).

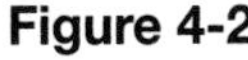

Figure 4-2

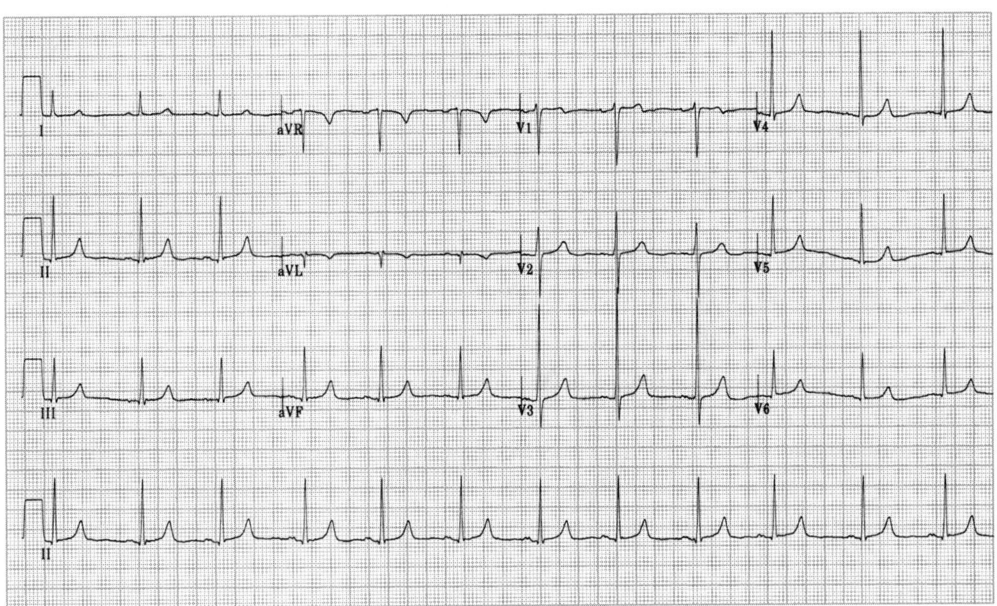

Figure 4-3

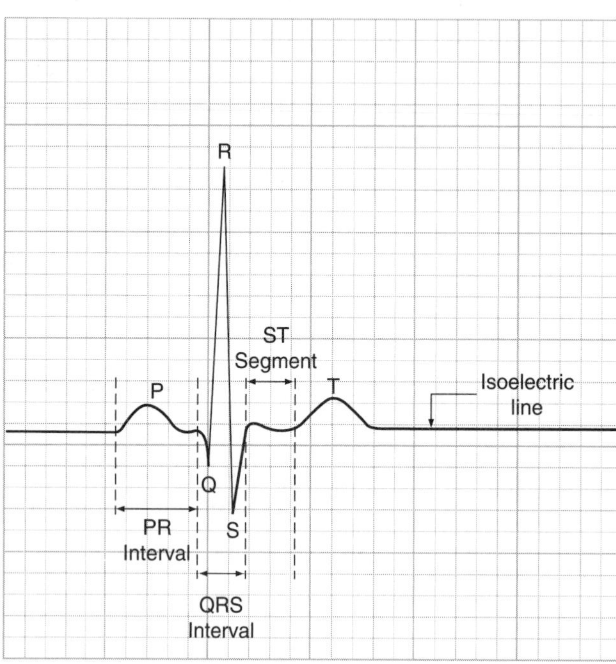

12-LEAD ECG INTERPRETATION

As mentioned earlier, the initial action is to evaluate the 3-lead rhythm strip (generally lead II or MCL 1) and address the rhythm or rate complications, which may cause cardiovascular instability. The 12-lead interpretation involves merely viewing the ST segment and its relationship to baseline—the isoelectric line (Figure 4-3).

While the QRS complex may be above or below the baseline (or both), the ST segment (the area from the end of the QRS to the beginning of the T-wave) should be even within the isoelectric line. This can be measured by placing a straightedge (like a piece of paper) horizontally along the isoelectric line just before the P-wave and running it straight through the complex to the ST segment; again, the beginning of the ST segment should be even with the isoelectric line at the beginning of the complex. Thus, the ST segment may be flat, elevated, or depressed in relation to the isoelectric baseline.

ST Segment Elevation

This is the cornerstone of 12-lead ECG identification (Figure 4-4). Elevation of greater than 1 mm (1 small box) in the patient with a cardiac event is indicative of acute myocardial infarction/myocardial *injury*. However, the myocardial muscle is salvageable if the coronary vessel can be reopened. In order for elevation to be a positive finding it must be present in two or

Figure 4-4 ST elevation

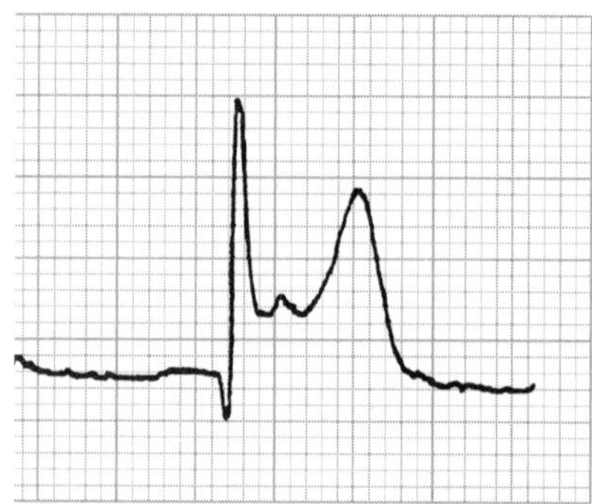

Figure 4-5 Normal 12-lead with left bundle branch block—unable to diagnose the ST segment

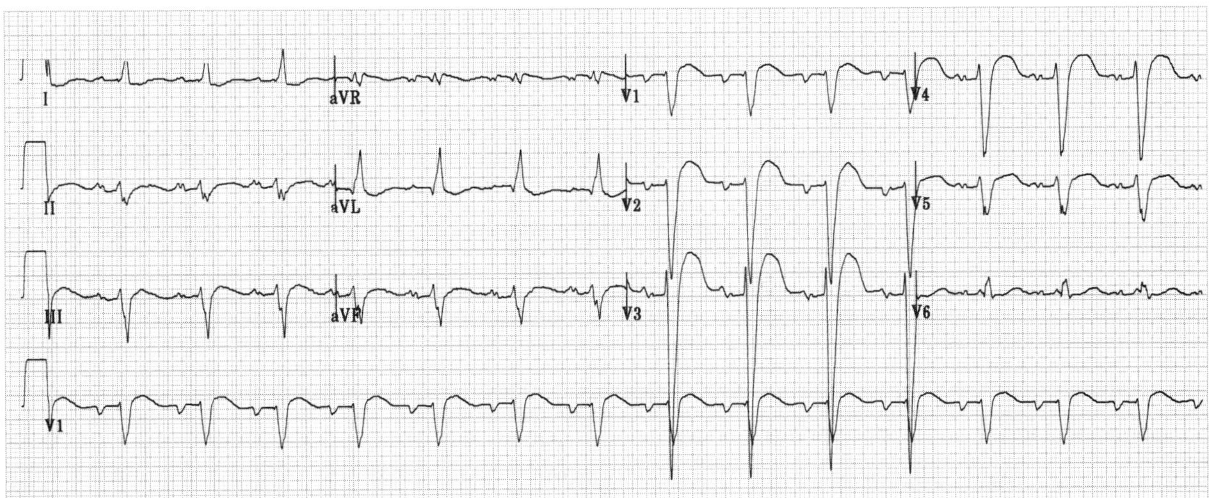

more contiguous leads (leads looking at the same area of the heart—refer back to the SALI acronym).

Following standard management with oxygen, aspirin, nitrates, pain control, and blood pressure control with beta blockers, the patient should be evaluated for fibrinolytics (medication) or percutaneous (mechanical) interventions such as angioplasty, stent, or coronary artery bypass grafting (CABG). This decision needs to be made emergently based on the capabilities of the team and facility currently managing the patient. The longer it takes to open the occluded vessel, the greater the chance becomes for cardiac arrest or cardiac complications such as congestive heart failure (CHF) or cardiogenic shock. In these cases, "Time is certainly muscle."

Also in the acute myocardial infarction criteria is the patient who presents with cardiac symptoms and a *new* left bundle branch block present on the 12-lead ECG.

The left bundle branch block is *diagnosed* by noting a QRS complex wider than 0.12 seconds (three small boxes) in the V1 lead (though all leads will show a wide QRS complex) with a negative (downward) QRS complex. The reason this is considered to be an acute infarction is an occlusion of the descending branch the left coronary artery (LAD) will cause blood flow to cease to the branches of the left-sided lower electrical pathways. Thus, a left bundle branch block occurs; this widens the QRS and makes the ST elevation difficult, if not impossible to diagnose (Figure 4-5). At this point it is assumed that patients with cardiac symptoms *and* a *new* left bundle branch block have suffered a recent AMI, and thus may be candidates for chemical or mechanical reperfusion therapy the same as the ST segment elevated AMI.

To an extent, right bundle branch blocks may present in a similar way but the ST segment can generally be evaluated and managed as appropriate.

It should be noted that several non-AMI conditions may also cause ST elevation, thus the patient and ECG must be evaluated by those skilled at 12-lead diagnosis. The following are some of the common "imposters" causing ST elevation: ventricular rhythms, pacemakers, left ventricular hypertrophy, coronary artery vasospasm, and early repolarization.

Figure 4-6 ST segment depression

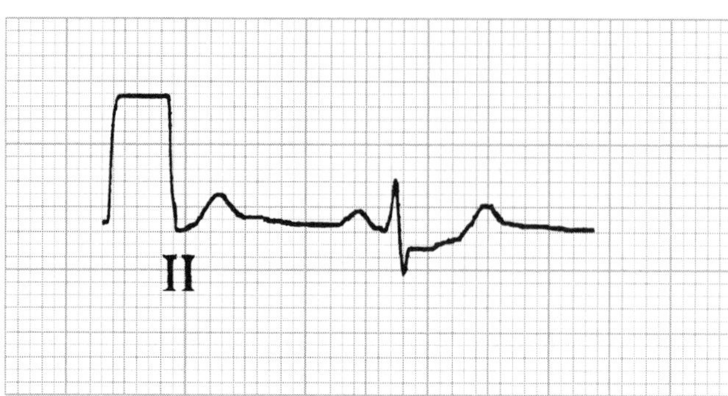

ST Segment Depression or Inverted T-Wave

ST depression is the term used as the T-wave begins while the ST segment has remained greater than 0.5 mm *below* the isoelectric baseline or the T-wave is simply flipped upside down. In the patient with cardiac symptoms this sign may indicate myocardial ischemia due to low oxygenated blood flow to the myocardium. This condition may be a bout of angina with no myocardial muscle damage or may be an early AMI where the myocardial muscle has not been injured enough to cause ST elevation...yet. Hence, ST depression and/or inverted T-waves require further investigation (Figures 4-6 and 4-7).

These ischemic changes require that the patient be continuously evaluated for a developing AMI; he should receive the standard O_2, nitrates, aspirin, and pain control along with some less aggressive "clot management" such as fractionated heparins and glycoprotein inhibitors. These patients are continually monitored and generally evaluated for cardiac catheterization, though not usually in the same rapid time frame as the ST elevated presents. However, it should be noted that patients with ST depression and other complications may be taken emergently for cardiac catheterization: angioplasty, stent, or coronary artery bypass grafting as needed.

Note: Inverted T-waves are normal in leads aVR and V1 if the QRS is negative and should not be addressed as a cardiac event in and of themselves.

Figure 4-7 T-wave inversion

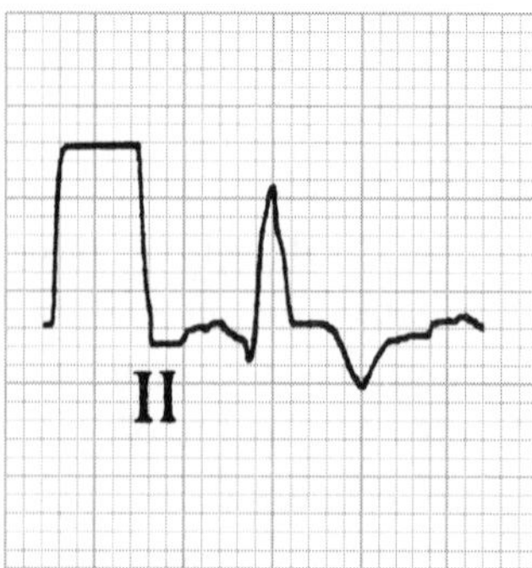

Q-Wave Development

The Q-wave occurs once the myocardial muscle has been deprived of oxygenated blood long enough for the muscle in that specific area to become necrotic (dead). This muscle section will not regenerate and will generally not "pump." These patients are prone to complications such as CHF and cardiogenic shock acutely and chronically without appropriate management. Though the coronary artery is occluded, the risk/benefit ratio of administering fibrinolytics to these patients is inappropriate as the muscle in the infarcted area is damaged beyond repair and opening the vessel will not change this fact. The transition from the injury phase (ST elevation) to the infarction phase with death of the myocardial muscle (Q-wave development) is based on the amount of time the coronary vessel is occluded and the muscle is deprived of oxygenated blood. The general management for these patients is to administer the standard cardiac medications as indicated by the patients' condition. These may include oxygen, aspirin, nitrates, pain control, fractionated heparin, and possibly glycoprotein inhibitors. These patients will generally end up in a diagnostic cardiac catheterization lab for angioplasty, stent, or CABG.

The Q-wave is recognized as a negative defection immediately following the P-wave. Small Q-waves may be normal, thus considered a physiological Q-wave. An abnormal (pathological) Q-wave is one in which the duration (width) is greater than 1 mm (1 small box) or the depth greater than one-third the height of the QRS complex (Figure 4-8).

Figure 4-8 Pathologic Q-wave

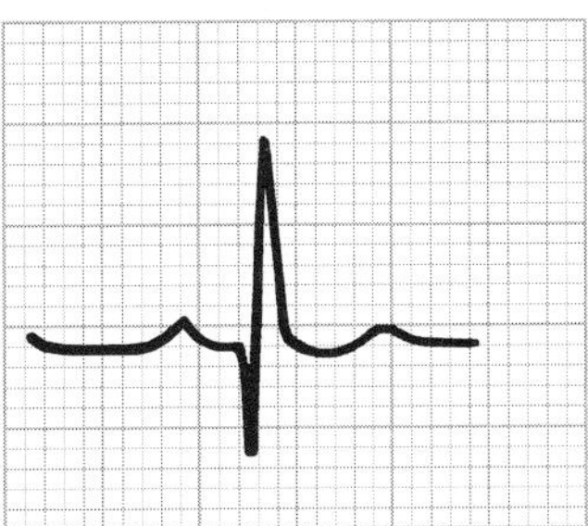

Figure 4-9 puts it all together.

Practice Test 12-Lead ECGs

Evaluate the following 12-lead ECGs for injury (ST elevation) or ischemia (ST depression or T-wave inversion). Then use the acronym SALI (page 69) to determine which area of the myocardium is being affected.

Figure 4-9

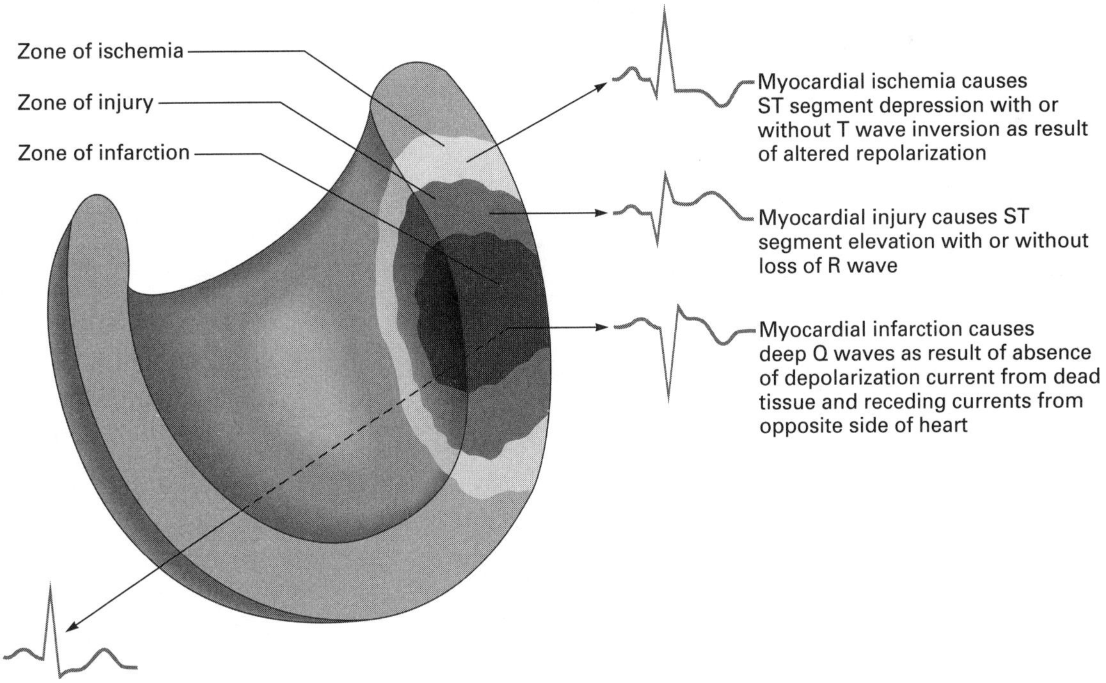

Zone of ischemia
Zone of injury
Zone of infarction
Myocardial ischemia causes ST segment depression with or without T wave inversion as result of altered repolarization
Myocardial injury causes ST segment elevation with or without loss of R wave
Myocardial infarction causes deep Q waves as result of absence of depolarization current from dead tissue and receding currents from opposite side of heart

1.

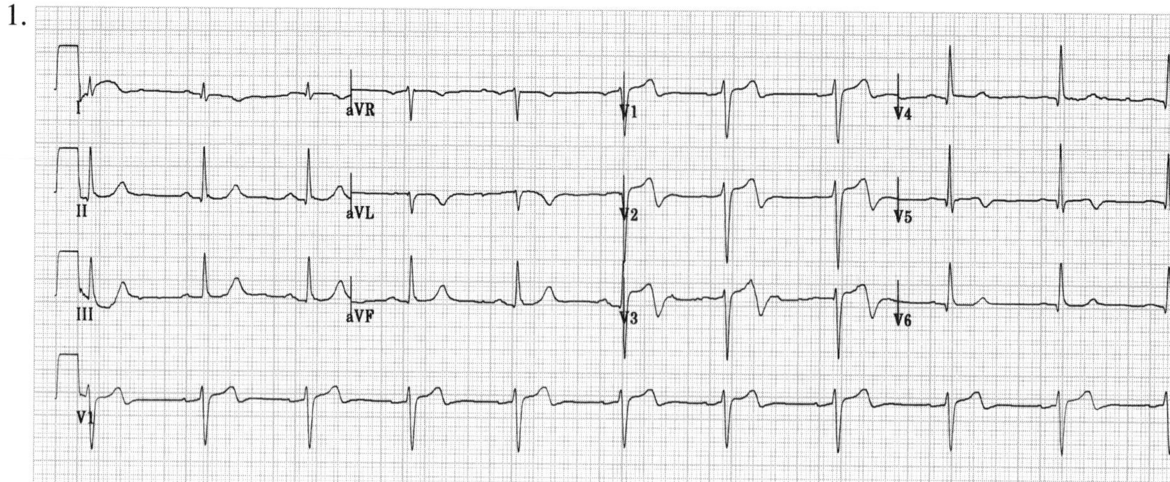
I
aVR
V1
V4
II
aVL
V2
V5
III
aVF
V3
V6
V1

2.

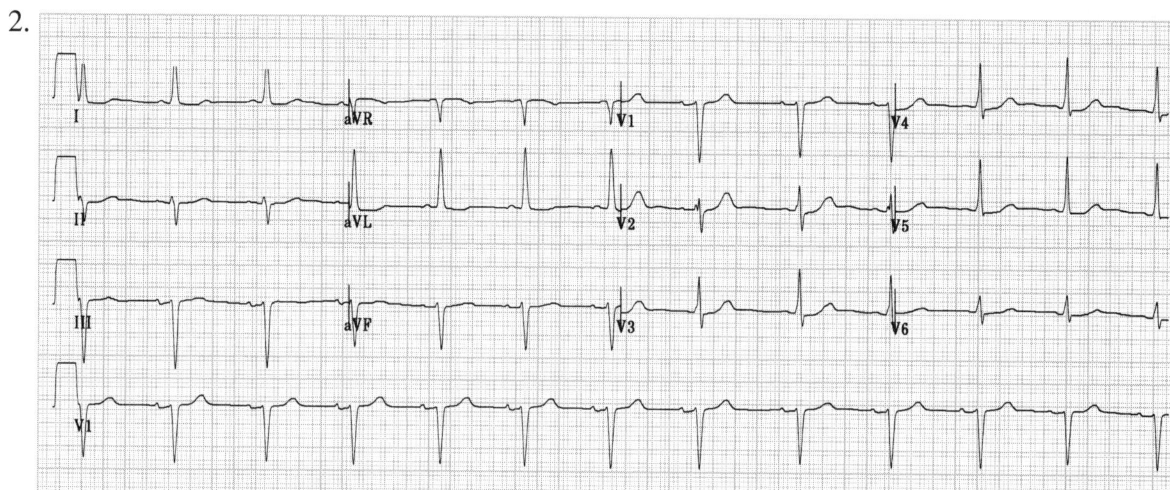
I
aVR
V1
V4
II
aVL
V2
V5
III
aVF
V3
V6
V1

3.

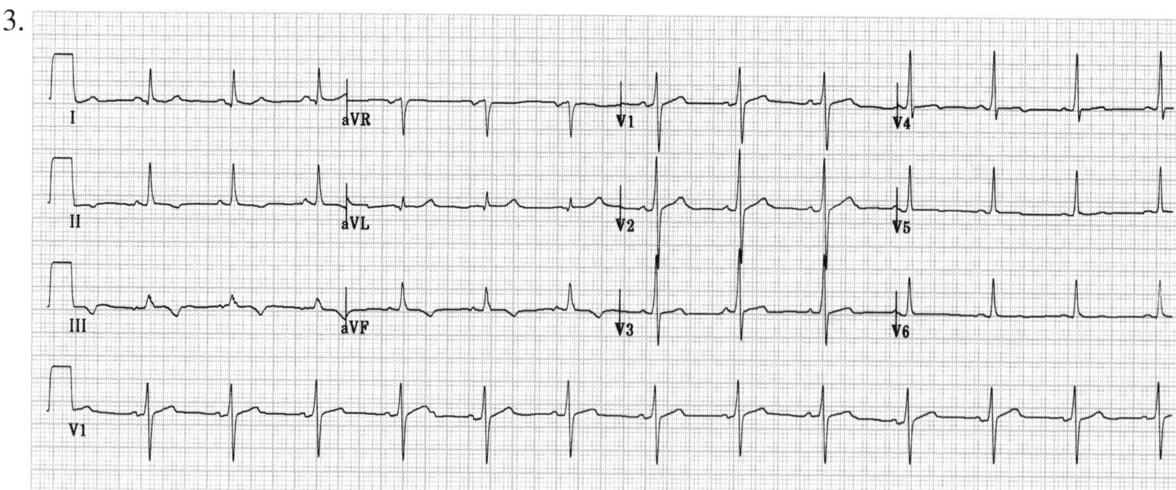
I
aVR
V1
V4
II
aVL
V2
V5
III
aVF
V3
V6
V1

4.

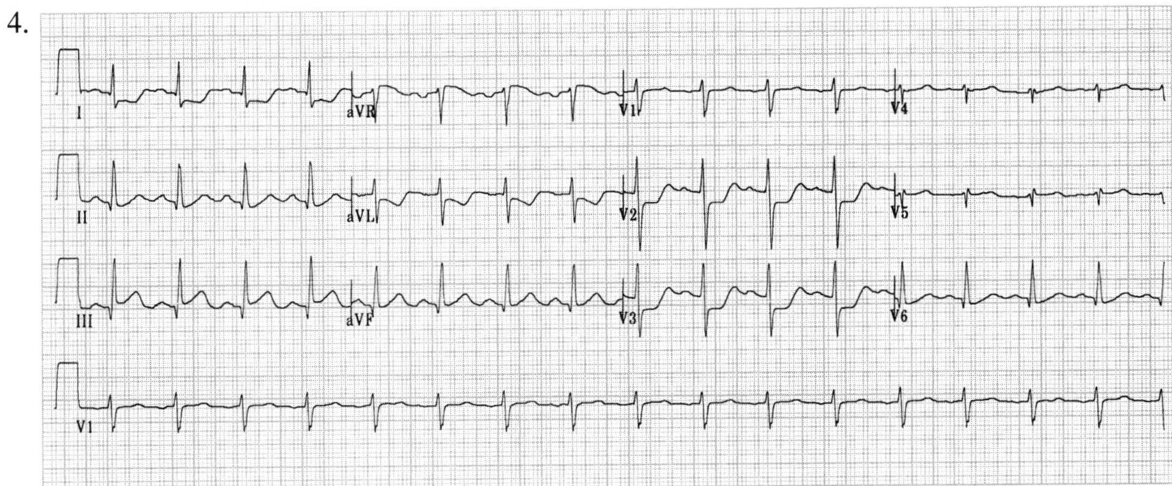

5.

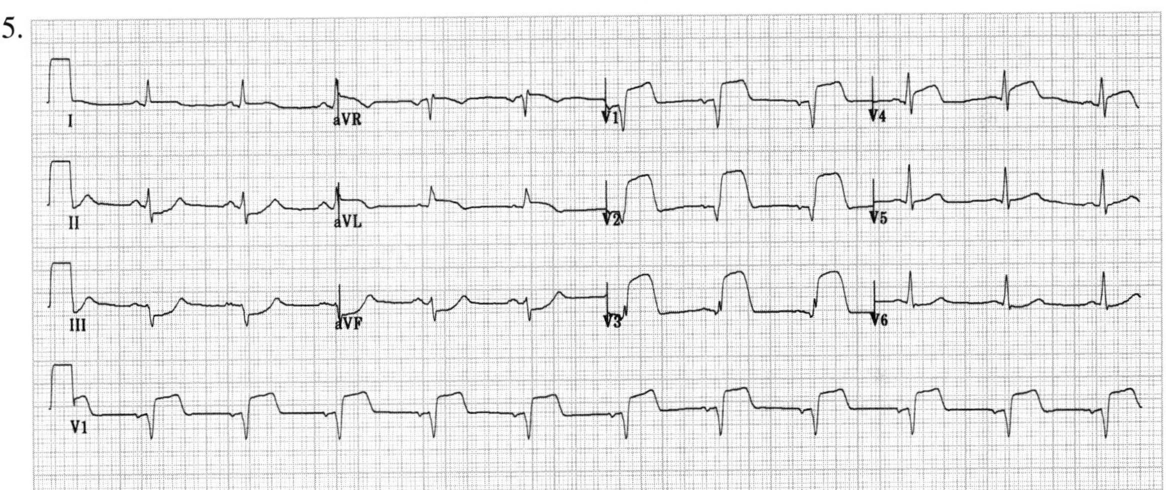

Again, this segment is merely a brief introduction to 12-Lead ECG evaluation. Patients should be managed based on their presenting symptoms, history, and clinical findings. The ECG should be evaluated by those skilled in interpretation and management should be based on ACLS guidelines and the clinical ability of the system or facility.

The key point is to recognize ECG irregularities, especially ST elevation, and have the patient managed by the appropriate team.

CHAPTER

5

Electrical Therapy

Why Electrical Therapy?

There are times when the patient's cardiac electrical activity is inappropriate. It may be too slow, too fast, or chaotic. The ACLS provider has the option to use electrical therapy—transcutaneous pacing, cardioversion, or defibrillation—to correct these electrical problems. Many providers will opt to use electrical therapy when there is an electricity versus medication decision to be made, due to the success rate of electrical therapies and the absence of unwanted side effects, medication interactions, and toxicity often associated with pharmacologic therapy.

Appropriate selection and utilization of these electrical therapies involves understanding indications, being familiar with the equipment, and feeling comfortable with each of the procedures.

Transcutaneous Pacing

Applications:

- Symptomatic bradycardia

Transcutaneous pacing is indicated in ACLS when a patient's heart rate is too slow, causing symptoms of poor oxygen delivery to important body systems (changes in mental status, low blood pressure, chest pain, pulmonary edema, cardiac arrest).

The transcutaneous (through the skin) pacemaker supplements the body's intrinsic pacemakers by delivering small amounts of electricity through the skin and smooth muscle to the myocardium. Once the impulse arrives at the heart, hopefully, excitability, conductivity, and contractility will take over and cause a faster heart rate, moving blood to where it needs to go.

Step 1: *Know your equipment.* The time to become familiar with your pacing equipment is well before you have a patient who is bradycardic, symptomatic, and in need of pacing. Prior to using the pacemaker, be sure you know the following about your equipment:

- Where is it located? If I need to pace a patient, do I go to my crash cart, somewhere else in my department, somewhere else in my facility?
- Where are the pacing pads kept? Are they already attached to the cable? In some drawer near the equipment?
- How do I attach the pacing cable to the monitor?
- How does the manufacturer of my equipment recommend I apply the pacing pads?
- How do I turn the pacemaker on?
- How do I set the rate?
- How do I increase the energy that flows through the pads (with button marked energy/output/mA/milliamps)?
- Do I have the ability to choose between fixed and demand mode?

Step 2: *Prepare yourself and the patient.* The prospect of any electricity flowing through one's chest can be frightening, so be sensitive to this when you explain the procedure to your patient. Also, be aware that pacing is uncomfortable for the patient. As the electricity from the pads passes through the skin, he will feel something like a bee sting 60 times a minute! As electricity passes through muscle, the muscle cells will contract, causing twitching. When preparing to pace, anticipate the potential need for sedation once the patient is more hemodynamically stable.

Step 3: *Apply the pads.* This type of pacing is achieved by placing pads on the skin (Figure 5-1). Two typical pad placements for pacer pads are anterior–anterior placement and anterior–posterior placement. Ensuring contact between the pads and the skin can maximize the chances that pacing will be effective. Remember to:

- Prepare the skin. Be sure it is clean and dry.
- Remove excess hair.
- Remove transdermal medication patches and wipe the area free of meds.

Figure 5-1a Applying ECG electrodes

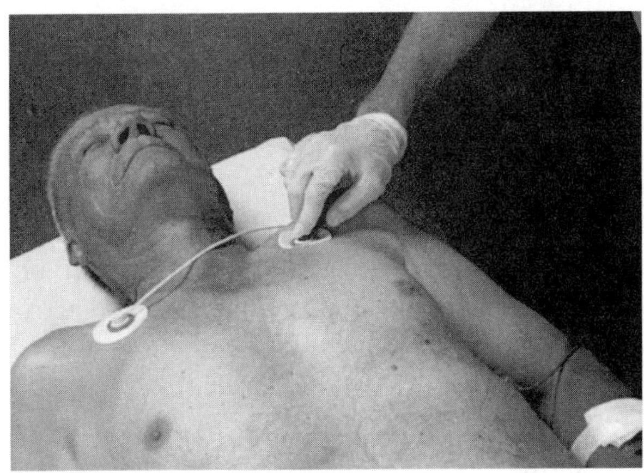

Figure 5-1b Applying pacing pads

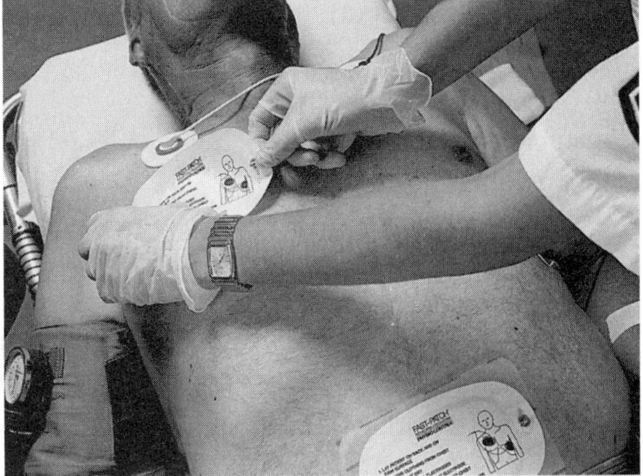

Figure 5-2 Select rate and current

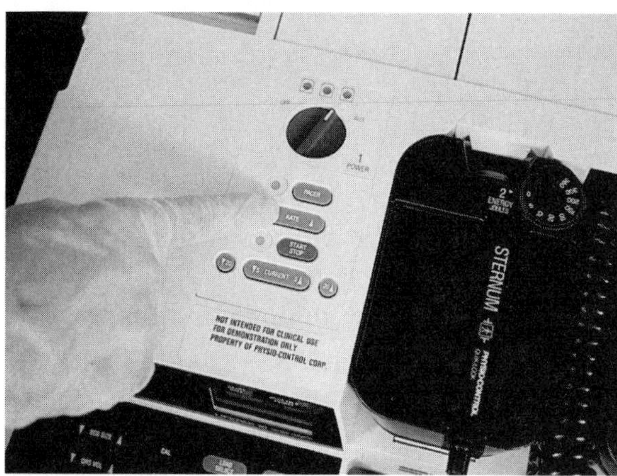

- Avoid implanted devices. If you see a pacemaker/defibrillator/infusion port under the skin, alter your pad placement slightly to avoid placing the pad over a device.

Also be sure that your patient is attached to the cardiac monitor via electrodes as well as the pacer pads. The electrodes will *receive* electrical impulses and translate them to the waveform on the monitor, while the pads will *send* the electrical impulses to stimulate the heart.

STEP 4: *Set the rate.* Set the pacemaker at a rate at 60 beats per minute (Figure 5-2). If pacing is successful, your patient's heart rate will be faster than bradycardia (which does a bad job of delivering blood), but slower than tachycardia (which increases myocardial oxygen demand and may decrease cardiac output).

STEP 5: *Pace.*

- Turn the pacemaker on.
- Increase the energy through the pads, while watching the monitor.
- Stop when you note electrical capture on the monitor (pacemaker spikes followed by a QRS complex), then increase by 10% more.
- Verify mechanical capture (check a pulse!).
- Reassess patient's hemodynamic status (check vital signs!). The rate may need to be increased above 60 if mentation and blood pressure are not adequte.
- Consider sedation if the patient is uncomfortable.

STEP 5: *Think about the long-term plan.*

- What is the cause of the patient's bradycardia, and can it be reversed?
- Will the patient need some other type of temporary pacing, such as transvenous pacing?
- Will the patient go to the operating room for implantable pacemaker?

Synchronized Cardioversion

Application:

- Unstable ventricular tachycardia (VT)
- Unstable supraventricular tachycardia (SVT).

Synchronized cardioversion is one procedure utilized to deliver an electrical shock to the heart muscle to depolarize the myocardium. Depolarizing heart cells all at once results in an electrical "time-out," stopping out-of-control electrical activity and allowing a more controlled pacemaker to take over.

In ACLS, synchronized cardioversion is indicated for patients with unstable tachycardias. Patients with significant changes in their mental status, blood pressure, development of chest pain, or pulmonary edema, as well as more subjective findings such as pallor, diaphoresis, or weakness may be considered unstable. The rationale for using electrical rather than drug therapy for the unstable patient is that cardioversion is considered more aggressive, may work more quickly, and involve fewer variables than pushing a medication. A patient who is showing signs of impaired perfusion to important body systems may need his tachycardia abolished immediately, rather than waiting for a medication to work.

Cardioversion differs from defibrillation in two ways:

- The energy delivered by cardioversion is initially lower than defibrillation.
- The energy is delivered more precisely, aimed at a particular phase of the QRS complex.

Think of cardioversion as an electrical bomb carefully aimed at the myocardium. We want the destruction of the arrhythmias to occur without too much damage.

STEP 1: *Know your equipment.* Being familiar with the equipment where you work will help you feel more confident and competent when the time comes to use it (Figure 5-3). Ask the following questions about the equipment that you would use to cardiovert.

- *Where is it located?* Cardioversion is usually one function of the monitor/defibrillator located with the emergency equipment available to healthcare personnel. Often the monitor is kept on or near the code cart (or crash cart) with emergency drugs and airway equipment.
- *Do I deliver the shock using pads or paddles?* Some equipment allows the user to choose between these two options. Know what is available to you. If using paddles, remember that you must also use some type of conductive medium (gel or paste) to enhance the conduction of electricity from the patient to the skin. You must also apply enough pressure on the paddles to flatten out the patient's curved chest against the flat paddles. If using self-adhesive pads, the conductive agent is built in and because the pads conform to the patient's chest, pressure is not needed. However, ensuring that the pads stick well to the chest is important, so excess hair, moisture, and medication patches should be removed before applying pads.

Figure 5-3a When cardioverting, be sure machine is set to "synch"

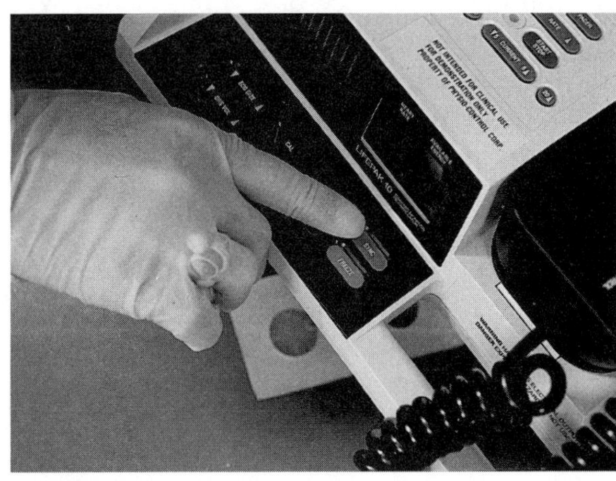

Figure 5-3b Apply paddles to patient's chest. Clear area before discharging paddles. Push buttons to discharge.

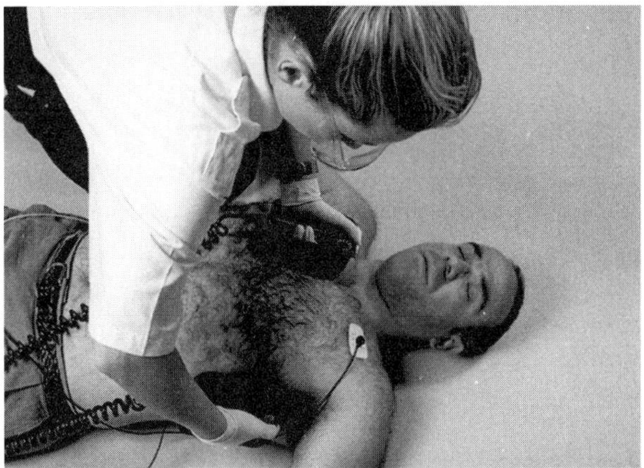

- *Where is the synchronize button?* Pressing this button is an important step in the cardioversion process, so know where it is.
- *How do I select the energy that will be delivered to the patient?* Find the button or dial that is used to choose how much electricity will flow through the paddles or pads.
- *How do I discharge the energy?* Find the buttons to make the paddles or pads "fire."

STEP 2: *Prepare yourself and the patient.*

- Be sure that the patient is being monitored on the same piece of equipment that will deliver the electricity. Use electrodes if you have paddles and put the pads on if you will use "hands off" therapy.
- Explain the procedure to the patient. Don't assume that someone with an altered mental status cannot hear you.
- Consider sedation. Cardioversion hurts! If the patient's mental status dictates, and his vital signs allow you to do so, consider that benzodiazapines may induce a bit of amnesia, and narcotics may provide some pain relief.
- Assemble appropriate people and equipment. Provide for privacy and safety.

STEP 3: *Cardiovert.*

- Apply pads or paddles.
- Press the synchronize button. Look for visual confirmation that your equipment is in the "synch" mode. The R-wave is usually marked and other visual cues, like lights or words on the screen, may indicate that your machine is ready to synchronize.
- Select the energy that you will deliver. Begin with 100 joules or the biphasic equivalent.
- Once the pads or paddles are charged, be sure everyone is clear. Make sure no one is touching the patient or anything that is touching the patient. Ensuring that nobody receives an accidental shock is your responsibility. Announce to everyone in the room something like: "On the count of three, I am going to shock. One, I'm clear (check yourself), two, you're clear (everyone else should check themselves), three, everybody's clear (visually sweep the room to be sure everyone is clear).
- Deliver the shock. Push the button(s) that discharge the pads or paddles. Hold them in until the electricity is discharged. This may not happen instantly, since the monitor will wait until the appropriate time in the QRS complex.

STEP 4: *Reevaluate.*

- Check the monitor. Has the rhythm changed?
- Check the patient. Is he still perfusing (is there a pulse)? Is he stable or unstable?
- If the patient remains tachycardic and unstable, repeat the procedure with the next highest energy setting. The sequence is 100, 200, 300, 360 joules, or the biphasic equivalent.
- If the patient's rhythm or status has changed, act accordingly.

Defibrillation

Applications:

- Ventricular fibrillation (VF)
- Pulseless ventricular tachycardia (VT)

Defibrillation is another procedure utilized to deliver an electrical shock to the heart muscle to depolarize the myocardium. Compared to cardioversion, defibrillation delivers a less precisely timed, larger shock to the myocardium.

Defibrillation, along with CPR, is a priority intervention for a patient in ventricular fib or pulseless ventricular tach. The sooner a well-oxygenated fibrillating heart is shocked, the better the chances of conversion to an organized electrical rhythm that may stimulate the heart to move blood around the body.

STEP 1: *Know your equipment.* Since the timeliness of defibrillation has such an impact on patient survival, knowing how to use the equipment before you are dealing with a cardiac arrest situation is critical (Figure 5-4). Ask the following questions about the equipment that you would use to defibrillate.

- *Where is it located?* Your monitor/defibrillator is probably located with the emergency equipment where you work. Often the monitor is kept on or near the code cart (crash cart) with emergency drugs and airway equipment.

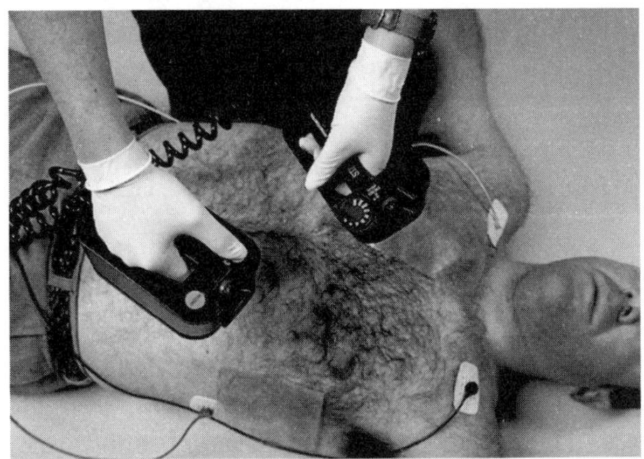

Figure 5-4a Apply paddles to chest

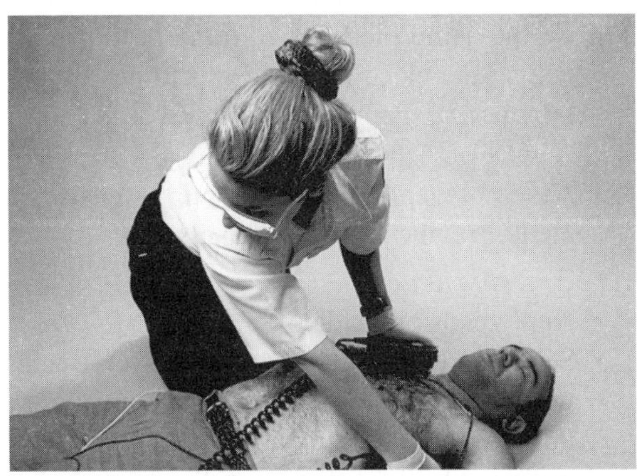

Figure 5-4c Reevaluate cardiac rhythm

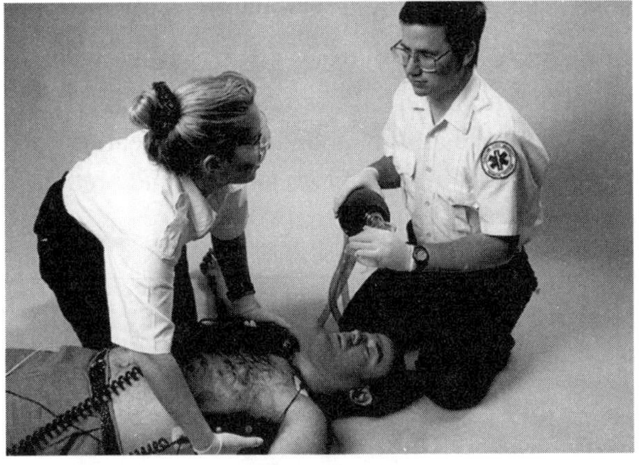

Figure 5-4b Clear people from around patient before delivering shock

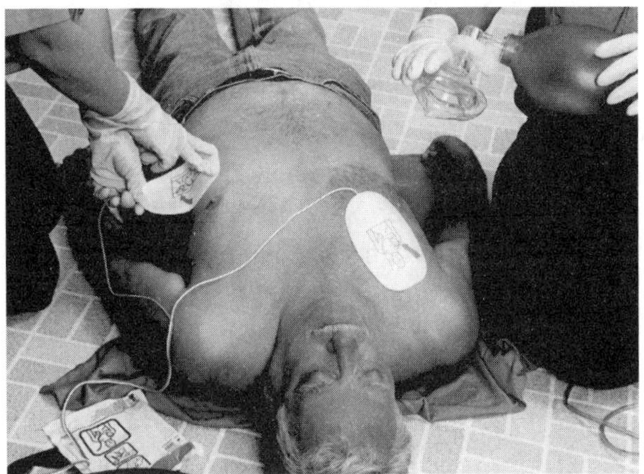

Figure 5-4d This procedure may be performed with hands-free pads

- *Is it plugged in when not in use?* Knowing if you should unplug the device before running to an emergency may help prevent your pulling a cart and leaving the monitor behind…crashing to the floor!
- *Do I deliver the shock using pads or paddles?* If using paddles, decrease the chest's resistance to energy by using conductive medium (gel or paste) and adequate paddle pressure. The built-in gel and aggressive adhesive minimize those concerns for users of hands-free pads. Don't forget to increase the chances of a good "stick" by removing excess hair or medication patches and making sure the skin is dry before applying pads.
- *How do I select the energy that will be delivered to the patient?* Find the button or dial that is used to choose how much electricity will flow through the paddles or pads.
- *How do I discharge the energy?* Find the buttons to make the paddles or pads "fire."

STEP 2: *Prepare yourself and the patient.*

- Be sure that the patient is being monitored on the same piece of equipment that will deliver the electricity. Use electrodes if you have paddles; put the pads on if you will use "hands-off" therapy.
- Assemble appropriate people and equipment. Provide for privacy and safety.

STEP 3: *Defibrillate.*

- Apply pads or paddles.
- Select the energy that you will deliver. Begin with 360 joules or the biphasic equivalent. Push the "charge" button. Listen for the monitor's auditory cue that it is fully charged.
- Be safety conscious! Before defibrillating the patient, make sure nobody is touching the patient. State "clear" loudly. Perform a visual sweep of the room.
- Deliver the shock. Push the button(s) that discharge the pads or paddles.

STEP 4: *Reevaluate.*

- Resume CPR immediately after the shock is delivered. After 2 minutes of CPR, check to see if the rhythm has changed and perfusion has been restored.
  - Check the patient. Does he have a pulse?
  - If the patient remains in ventricular fibrillation or pulseless ventricular tachycardia, repeat the procedure.
- If the patient's rhythm or status has changed, act accordingly.

Quick Tip

Monophasic or biphasic: Which is better?

The terms *monophasic* and *biphasic* refer to the direction that electricity travels when a shock is delivered through various brands of equipment. The experts are reluctant to declare that one method is superior, since there are studies to support the use of monophasic as well as high-energy and low-energy biphasic defibrillators. The bottom line: Be familiar with the equipment available where you practice. Follow manufacturer's recommendations regarding energy selection. Do it quickly! The critical point is delivering a defibrillatory shock in a timely manner.

Automated External Defibrillation

An automated external defibrillator (AED) may be used in settings where manual defibrillators are not available, personnel do not interpret arrhythmias, or where the first responder to an emergency may not be a medically trained person (Figure 5-5).

The difference between a manual defibrillator and an AED is that the automated defibrillator will analyze a heart rhythm and deliver a shock if necessary, without decision-making on the operator's part. In the event that you need to use an AED, the steps are easy and begin with the steps of CPR:

- Assess for responsiveness. If an individual is unresponsive, call for help and get the AED.
- Open the airway and check for breathing. If no breathing, give two slow rescue breaths.

Figure 5-5a Monophasic Lifepack 500 AED

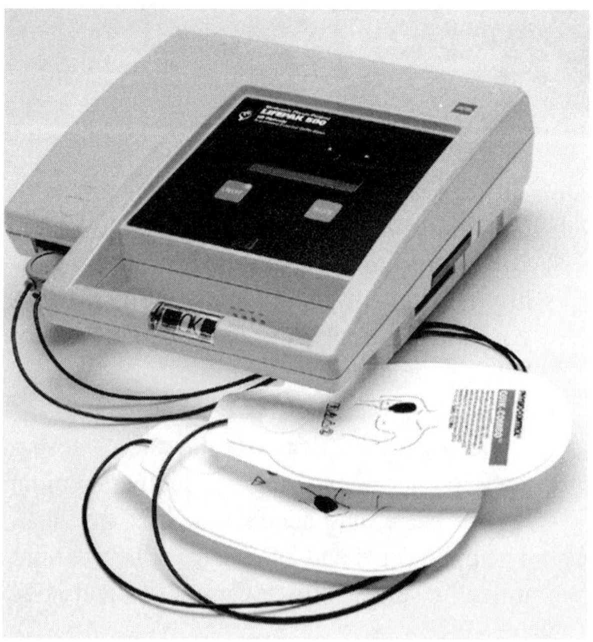

Figure 5-5b Biphasic Powerheart AED

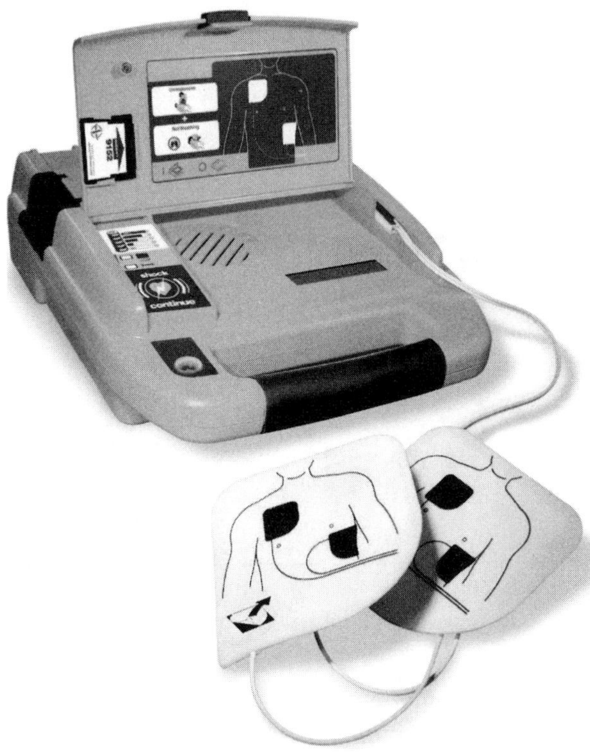

- Check for a pulse. If no pulse, begin chest compressions and the 30:2 compression to ventilation ratio until the AED arrives.
- As soon as the AED is available, open the device if there is a cover, and turn it on.
- Follow the voice prompts to apply pads to the patient's bare chest. Refer to pictures on the device or the pads if you are unsure about pad placement.
- Allow the device to analyze the patient's heart rhythm. During the analyze phase of operation, do not touch the patient. Stop compressions and ventilations and avoid making any motion, which could cause the machine to stop the analysis.
- If a shock is indicated, the machine will instruct you to stand clear and push a specific button to shock. Use the same procedure to clear the patient as you do prior to shocking with a manual defibrillator.
- After the shock is delivered, resume CPR. After 2 minutes of CPR, check for a pulse and allow the AED to analyze the patient's rhythm again.
- If the patient regains a pulse or respirations, place the patient in the recovery position and leave the AED pads on the patient until help arrives.
- If the machine reports that no shock is advised, then reassess the patient and begin CPR if the patient is not breathing and has no pulse. Leave the machine turned on and connected to the patient for follow-up rhythm analysis.
- When EMS personnel arrive, report what has been happening and allow them to assume control of the patient and equipment.

CHAPTER

6 Pharmacology Overview

Please note: The following psychomotor skills are discussed globally and generically as to their exact technique. An ACLS course does not provide licensure or certification to perform a specific skill. Practitioners who are authorized to perform such skills in their professional role must follow the guidelines and procedures set forth by their experience, clinical setting, or local policy.

Management of patients with acute coronary syndromes, cardiac arrest, and postarrest management all require intravenous (IV) access. Choosing the appropriate IV site will allow for a medication and fluid route, the ability to draw blood for laboratory studies, and when necessary, the ability to access the central circulation for more effective medication delivery, the ability to "insert" a transvenous pacemaker, and to perform advanced cardiovascular monitoring.

Peripheral IVs

Peripheral IVs are the most common access sites initially obtained in most patients (Figure 6-1). The standard fluid for patients who are not in cardiac arrest will depend on the patient's history, condition, and physician preference. In general, cardiac arrest victims should not receive IV fluids containing glucose as the extra administration of glucose may have a negative effect on neurologic recovery. Thus, the standard fluid used during cardiac arrest is sodium chloride or lactated ringers. These fluids also have the ability to

Figure 6-1 Peripheral IV sites

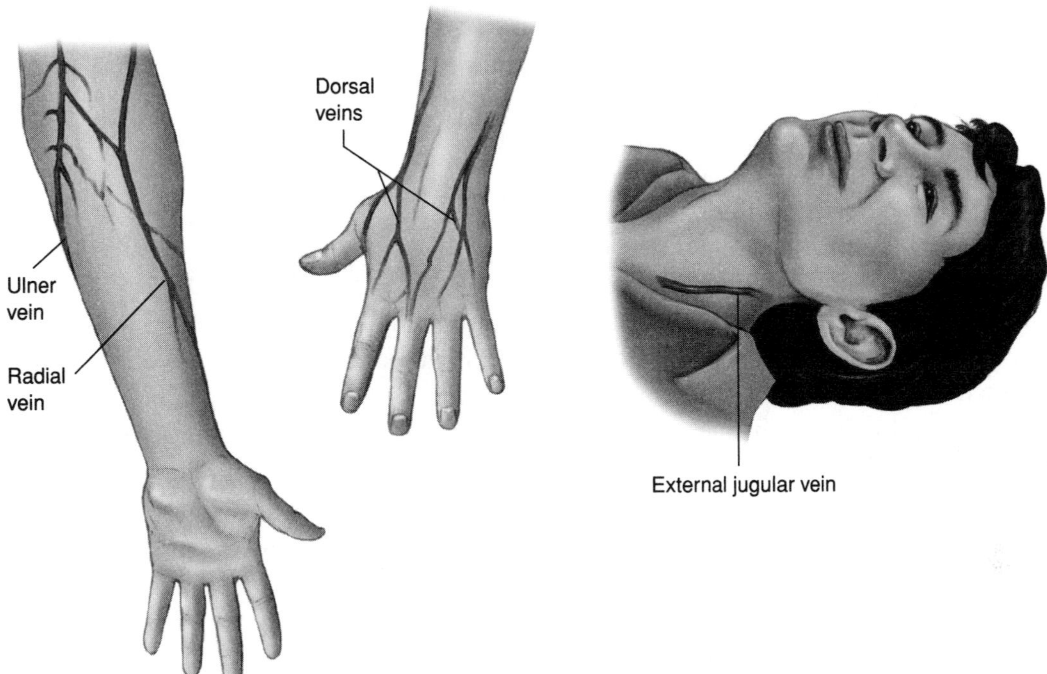

remain in the vascular space longer than dextrose, thus they may be used to increase circulating volume (as a fluid bolus) and may help move medications though the vascular space more readily. In patients who are not in profound hypoperfused or cardiac arrest states, a standard sized 22-18 gauge over the needle catheter in the hand or arm will suffice initially. For patients in poor circulation states including cardiac arrest, the preferred catheter is a large bore 18-14 gauge in a large vein such as the antecubital or external jugular vein. Peripheral sites are often relatively easy to establish, can be performed without stopping CPR, and generally do not cause significant complications, such as bleeding, or interference with circulation if the attempt is not successful. Disadvantages related to peripheral IV sites include the fact that they may be difficult to access in the cardiac arrest state and the medication distribution is slow (1–2 minutes) in cardiac arrest. The recommended procedure to follow when establishing and utilizing IV access in cardiac arrested patients is to attempt to utilize large veins in the upper arm with the largest catheter the provider is comfortable establishing, elevating the extremity after medication administration, flushing the medication with 20 cc of IV fluid, and performing CPR for up to 2 minutes after each medication before moving to the next drug. As with any invasive vascular procedure IVs run the risk of causing phlebitis or infection locally or systemically, thus, aseptic technique during placement is required. Though minimal, IVs do run the risk of air embolism, or catheter shear.

Intraosseous (IO) Access

Placing a needle into the bone marrow cavity is a procedure that has been utilized since World War II. The skill has been taught extensively in pediatric emergency courses since the 1990s. During the 2000s several adult devices have been utilized and studied, and have gained acceptance. The results have been positive: a bone marrow aspirating type needle (a needle with a removable inner stylette) can be placed into the bone marrow cavity (currently the tibia, humerus, or upper sternum) and fluids or medications infused with nearly the same absorption reliability as a peripheral IV site (Figure 6-2). The obvious advantage is this allows for rapid access with reliable flow in patients for whom IV access is not obtainable; hence, the indication for utilizing the intraosseous procedure is the need for emergency vascular access where a peripheral IV site is not available or unsuccessful. Of the devices currently available one type is manually inserted in a twisting fashion, two are spring loaded, and one utilizes a small drill. While each device has its own particular design uses and contraindications, the general rule is not to place the needle in a bone that is fractured, burned or infected. The use of these devices is relatively easy; however, like all procedures the provider must be trained, skilled, and authorized to utilize an intraosseous device. Studies in 2005 recommend IO access over tracheal administration of medications for emergency access when an IV is unavailable.

Central Venous Access

Establishing central venous access is indicated in critical patients for whom IV access has been unsuccessful or is not possible. Central lines may also be placed in patients who are going to require long-term or continuous vascular access. Access to the central circulation (vena cava, right atrium, and pulmonary artery) via a peripheral

Figure 6-2a Intraosseous needle in place

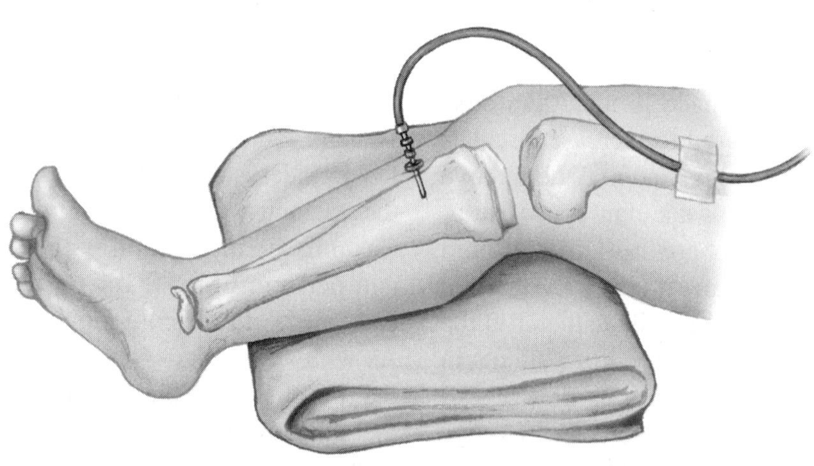

Figure 6-2b Manual intraosseous needle

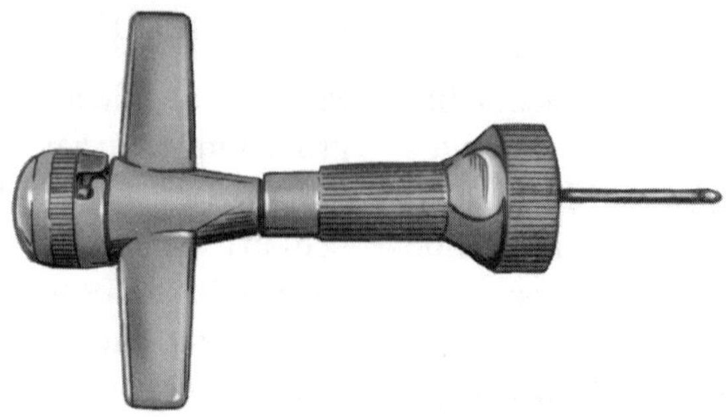

vein and long catheter utilized to place a transvenous pacemaker and advanced central pressure monitoring devices is also possible. Certainly administering medications directly into the central circulation during cardiac arrest is superior to the peripheral or intraosseous routes; however, unless the central line is already in place, this procedure may be too labor intensive and time consuming to use as a "first attempt." Central venous access is a quasi-surgical procedure that requires a sterile field, an extremely skilled and authorized provider and assistants who are familiar with the device and kit utilized to place the line. The most common sites used are the subclavian vein, internal jugular vein (both of which require CPR to be halted), and the femoral vein. These are large predictable sites, which will allow for rapid flow once established. Some disadvantages of central lines include: the skill level required limits this to mainly advanced critical care providers, the potential to create a pneumothorax or hematoma that compromises the airway, and the contraindication to the use of fibrinolytics should the patient be a candidate. Central lines also have a greater potential for infection, air embolism, and catheter shear. So while central lines do provide for better flow and absorption of medications, the skill level and subset of providers authorized and proficient at placing them during a cardiac arrest are such that most standard ACLS courses do not specifically teach the psychomotor skill of placing a central line during cardiac arrest. It should be noted in the setting where a patient does have a central venous catheter in place or if one is inserted during the course of treatment, the delivery of fluids and medications via this site is superior (Figure 6-3).

Figure 6-3 Central venous catheter

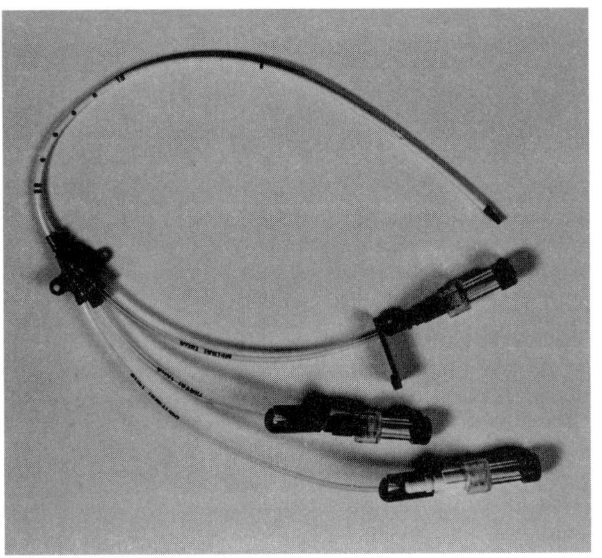

Pharmacology Overview

After close review of all scientific evidence available, most experts acknowledge that there are very few drugs whose use in cardiac arrest and prearrest arrhythmias is well supported. Therefore, in cardiac arrest, medication use is secondary to other interventions. Rescuers must place priority on basic CPR, defibrillation if appropriate, airway management, and then intravenous access and the use of appropriate drugs.

Despite the decreased role of pharmacology in cardiac arrest management, it remains critical that the provider not only rapidly recall appropriate drugs and dosages, but also demonstrate an in-depth knowledge of the medication action, indications, contraindications, and side effects.

ACLS pharmacology is divided into two categories. *Pharmacology I* encompasses agents used for patients in cardiac arrest or significant arrhythmias. *Pharmacology II* agents are used during the postresuscitation phase, and to treat acute coronary syndromes.

This overview is not intended to give all the possible options for dosages or usages, nor is it intended to be a substitute for reading and understanding the pharmacology section of your ACLS text.

Remember this about giving medications during cardiac arrest:

- Give medications via a large bore IV catheter (the bigger the better given available options).
- Locate the IV site fairly close to the heart. The antecubital fossa and the external jugular vein are two large conveniently located sites.
- Hang normal saline or lactated ringers solution with macro drip tubing.
- Each medication should be followed by at least 20 cc of the flush.
- Elevate the extremity to allow gravity to assist with delivery of the drug (don't dislodge the IV catheter!).
- Follow each medication dose with 2 minutes of CPR to circulate the drug.
- Reassess rhythm and pulses after each intervention.

Quick Tip

Remember the acronym NAVEL.

If no IV or I/O site is available, the following medications can be given through the ET tube:

- Narcan
- Atropine
- Vasopressin
- Epinephrine
- Lidocaine
  - Pass a catheter beyond the tip of the tracheal tube.
  - Administer 2–2.5 times the IV dose (vasopressin may be used at the IV dose).
  - Dilute the drug in 10 cc of NS or distilled water (if it is not packaged in 10 cc).
  - Stop compressions before you administer anything down the tube.
  - Administer the medication down the tube.
  - Spray the drug quickly down the catheter.
  - Deliver several breaths with the bag valve mask.
  - Resume CPR to circulate the drug.
  - Make sure the needles or needleless catheters are firmly attached to or removed from the syringe prior to administering the drug into the tracheal tube or catheter.

Learning the details of ACLS medications—drug, indications, dose, route, special considerations—can be a time-consuming and daunting task. However, understanding how the medications work and why they are used contribute to learning and retaining this material, rather than the mere memorization that may get you through an exam but may not help months later in a clinical situation.

For easy reference, the medications here are presented in alphabetical order. It may be easier to learn the medications, however, if you classify them according to action or indications:

ANTIARRHYTHMICS

Rhythm Control	*Rate Control*
Lidocaine	Calcium channel blockers
Amiodarone	Diltiazem
Procainamide	Verapamil
Magnesium	Adenosine
Ibutilide	Digitalis

MEDICATIONS FOR ACUTE CORONARY SYNDROMES

Aspirin

Nitroglycerine

Morphine

Beta blockers

Anticoagulants

Fibrinolytics

Heparin

- Unfractionated
- Fractionated

Clopidogrel

Glycoprotein IIb/IIIa inhibitors

ACE inhibitors

MEDICATIONS TO TREAT HYPOTENSION

Dopamine

Norepinephrine

Dobutamine

MEDICATIONS TO TREAT PULMONARY EDEMA

Nitroglycerine

Nitroprusside

Furosemide

Morphine

VASOPRESSORS IN CARDIAC ARREST

Vasopressin

Epinephrine

MEDICATIONS TO TREAT SPECIFIC ARRESTS

Magnesium

Calcium chloride

Sodium bicarbonate

REVERSAL AGENTS

Flumazenil

Naloxone

ACE Inhibitors

Enalapril (Vasotec), Captopril (Capoten), Lisinopril (Prinivil)

Classification

Antihypertensive

Indications

- Hypertension
- CHF
- Post-MI

Action

- Selectively suppresses the renin-angiotensin-aldosterone system
- Inhibits the conversion of angiotensin I-angiotensin II, resulting in dilation of arterial and venous vessels
- Attenuates cardiac remodeling post-MI

Dosage

Vasotec: 5–40 mg po qd, 0.625–1.25 mg IV over 5 min q6hr

- Capoten: 12.5–50 mg po bid/tid
- Prinivil: 10–40 mg po qd

Route

IV, po

Side effects

Hypotension, chest pain, tachycardia, arrhythmias

Adenosine

Adenocard

Classification

Antiarrhythmic

Indications

Narrow complex tachycardia due to reentry

Actions

Abolishes reentry, slows AV conduction

Dosage

6 mg IV/IO rapidly over 1–3 seconds, followed by saline flush, 20 cc. May be repeated at 12 mg rapid IV/IO × 2

Route

IV/IO push-rapid (Adenosine has a 10–30-second half-life)

Consideration

- Transient reentry arrhythmias, chest pain, palpitations, flushing, headache are common following administration
- Will not convert atrial fibrillation or atrial flutter

Quick Tip

Give this drug as rapidly as possible. Put the drug in the injection port closest to the patient and the flush in the next distal port. Close the IV clamp, and push drug…follow with flush…fast!

Amiodarone

Cordarone

Classification

Antiarrhythmic

Indications

- After defibrillation and pressor in cardiac arrest with persistent VT or VF
- Stable VT
- Ventricular rate control of rapid atrial arrhythmias in patients with severe LV dysfunction
- Control of hemodynamically stable VT or polymorphic VT, or wide complex tachycardia of unknown origin

Actions

- Prolongs the recovery period of cardiac cells after they have carried an impulse
- Effects sodium, potassium, and calcium channels and α and β channels
- Has greater efficacy and lower incidence of proarrhythmic properties than other drugs in patients with severely impaired heart function

Dosage

- VF/VT-cardiac arrest: 300 mg IV/IO in 20-30 cc D5W, may repeat × 1 @ 150 mg
- Perfusing patients: Rapid infusion 150 mg IV over 10 min, followed by infusion

Route

IV/IO

Considerations

- Hypotension, bradycardia may be associated with multiple dosing
- Medication has long half-life

Infusion

900 mg/500 cc (1.8 mg/cc)

Infuse @ 33 cc/hr × 6 hr (slow infusion—1 mg/min), then 17 cc/hr (maintenance infusion—0.5 mg/min) for 18 hr

Quick Tip

Some manufacturers of Amiodarone package the drug diluted in a carrier solution that foams when agitated. Draw up slowly and avoid shaking the drug vial.

Aspirin

Classifications

Anticoagulant, antipyretic, analgesic

Indications

Any patient with symptoms suggestive of myocardial ischemia. Acute MI and unstable angina

Actions

Blocks formation of thromboxin A_2, which is responsible for platelet aggregation and vasoconstriction, thus keeping platelets from becoming lodged in partially occluded coronary vessels

Dosage

162–325 mg chewable tablets. For patients unable to take po meds, may use rectal suppository 300 mg

Atropine

Classification

Parasympatholytic (blocks acetylcholine from the parasympathetic nervous system)

Indications

- Symptomatic bradycardia
- Asystole

Action

Increases heart rate and conduction through the AV node

Dosage

0.5 mg IV/IO for perfusing patients, 1.0 mg IV/IO in cardiac arrest. Repeat at 5-minute intervals if needed. Maximum total dose 3 mg or 0.04 mg/kg.

Considerations

- Tachycardia may result, so use in caution in the setting of ACS (Acute Coronary Syndrome).
- Smaller doses than 0.5 mg may cause bradycardia.

Quick Tip

"Give 0.5 if alive." Minimize the possibility of tachycardia in perfusing patients.

Beta Blockers

Metoprolol, Atenolol, Esmolol

Classification

Beta adrenergic blocker

Indications

- Suspected MI/unstable angina, to decrease oxygen consumption
- May be used prophylactically following an MI to reduce oxygen consumption

Actions

Decreases heart rate, stroke volume, contractility, decreasing oxygen demand

Dosage

- Metoprolol (Lopressor): 5 mg IV; may repeat in 5 min to max of 15 mg
- Atenolol (Tenormin): 5 mg over 5 min; may repeat in 10 min
- Esmolol (Brevibloc): 0.5 mg/kg over 1 min
- Labetalol: 10 mg IV/IO over 1–2 min. May repeat q 10 min

Side effects

Bradycardia, hypotension, bronchospasm

Calcium

Calcium chloride, Calcium gluconate

Classification

Calcium ion (electrolyte)

Indications *(should not be administered unless these conditions exist):*

- Hypocalcemia
- Hyperkalemia
- Calcium channel blocker overdose/adverse effect

Actions

Increased inotropic effect, increased automaticity

Dosage

- *Calcium chloride:* 2–4 mg/kg IV/IO of a 10% solution repeated in 10 min if necessary (may give as much as 8–16 mg/kg for hyperkalemia or calcium channel blocker OD)
- *Calcium gluconate:* 5–8 ml IV/IO

Considerations

- Ensure that IV tubing is well flushed before and after administration (will precipitate if mixed with sodium bicarb)
- May precipitate digitalis toxicity

Clopidogrel

Plavix

Classification

Anticoagulant

Indications

- High risk ST depression or T-wave inversion
- Patients with planned PCI
- Antiplatelet therapy in patients who cannot take aspirin

Actions

Inhibits platelet aggregation

Dosage

300 mg po initially, followed by 75 mg po qd

Considerations

- Caution in patients with history of bleeding; contraindicated in patients actively bleeding
- Metabolized by the liver—use caution in patients with impaired hepatic function
- Do not administer if cardiac surgery planned in the near future

Digitalis

Lanoxin, Digoxin

Classification

Cardiac glycoside

Indications

- CHF (better for chronic management than acute)
- Chronic atrial fibrillation

Actions

- Increases stroke volume by increasing force of contraction
- Slows conduction through the AV node

Dosage

Loading dose: 10–15 μg/kg lean body weight (usually 0.5–1.0 mg)

Maintenance dose is determined by patient's size, renal function, and blood levels

Considerations

Interacts with Amiodarone. Use ½ Digoxin dose when patient taking Amiodarone

Diltiazem HCL

Cardizem

Classification

Antiarrhythmic (calcium channel antagonists)

Indications

Supraventricular tachyarrhythmias

Actions

- Calcium channel antagonist
- Slows conduction
- Smooth muscle dilation

Dosage

- 15–20 mg (0.25 mg/kg) IV/IO over 2 minutes, may repeat with 25 mg IVP in 15 minutes if needed
- Infusion: mix 1:1 (e.g.: 125 mg/100 cc) infuse at 5–15 mg/hr

Route

IV push slowly and IV infusion

Side effects

Bradycardia, hypotension

Quick Tip

Reverse calcium channel blocker adverse effects with IV fluids, epinephrine infusion or pacing to increase heart rate, and calcium administration.

Dobutamine

Dobutrex

Classification

Adrenergic stimulator (used to increase cardiac output)

Indications

- SBP 70–100 mm Hg without signs of shock in patients with pump problems:
  - CHF
  - Pulmonary edema

Actions

Primarily beta effects causing a selective increase in stroke volume without a substantial increase in heart rate. (Lower doses are less likely to cause tachycardia and increased O_2 demand than dopamine.)

Dosage

Mix 500 mg/250 cc D5W = 2000 μg/cc. Infuse at 2–20 μg/kg/min (average patient to start at approximately 4 cc/hr)

Route

IV infusion only

Side effects

Tachycardia, chest pain, palpitations, increased O_2 demand if HR is increased.

Dopamine

Classification

Adrenergic stimulator (sympathetic nervous system)

Indications

- Symptomatic hypotension
- Refractory bradycardia

Actions

- Dopaminergic effects (1–2 μg/kg/min): Dilation of renal and mesenteric arteries
- Beta effects (2–10 μg/kg/min): Primarily increased heart rate and force increasing cardiac output
- Alpha effects (10–20 μg/kg/min): Peripheral vasoconstriction, increasing afterload

Dosage

2–20 μg/kg/min (usual cardiac starting dose 5 μg/kg/min)

Mix 400 mg/250 cc D5W = 1600 μg/cc. Begin at 5 μg/kg/min and titrate to a systolic BP 90 mm Hg.

Initial drip rate to infuse 5 μg/kg/min = 10% of patient's weight in pounds

Example: 150 lb patient: Rate = 15 cc/hr, 90 lb patient: Rate = 9 cc/hr

Route

IV infusion only

Side effects

Chest pain, tachyarrhythmias, PVCs

Quick Tip

Consider adding fluid volume when administering an inotropic agent if the patient may be hypovolemic. Remember Starling's law: "You need stretch of the muscle before you get squeeze."

Epinephrine

Classification

Adrenergic (sympathetic) stimulator

Indications

- Cardiac arrest
- Symptomatic bradycardia refractory to atropine, transcutaneous pacing, and dopamine

Actions

- Positive β effects, including increased heart rate, contractility, and automaticity
- Positive α effects, including peripheral vasoconstriction

Dosage

- Bolus: 1 mg IV/IO q 3–5 min, may use higher doses for bradycardic arrests caused by overdoses of agents such as calcium channel blockers or beta blockers
- Infusion: Mix 2 mg/500 cc D5W or NS. Infuse 1–10 μg/min

Route

IV/IO, ET, IV infusion

Adverse effects

Tachycardia, hypertension, PVCs, palpitations, increased myocardial O_2 demand

Fibrinolytics

Antistreplase, Alteplase, Reteplase, Tenekteplase

Classification

Fibrinolytic

Indications

- AMI less than 12 hours old with 12-lead ECG showing ST elevation in two related leads
- AMI less than 12 hours old with 12-lead ECG showing new bundle branch block
- Acute ischemic stroke of less than 3 hours with no bleed on CT scan

Actions

- Lysis of fibrin, which holds together thrombi blocking coronary or cerebral arteries
- Decrease in thrombus size allows enhanced blood flow distal to the clot

Dosage

- *Reteplase* (Retavase): 10 units IV followed by a 10 unit bolus 30 min apart
- *Alteplase* (Activase-TpA): 15 mg IV bolus, then 0.75 mg/kg over 30 min, then 0.5 mg/kg over 60 min
- *Activase for stroke:* 0.9 mg/kg (max. 90 mg) 10% as bolus and remaining over 60 min
- *Tenectaplase:* Single bolus 30–50 mg (depending on weight) IVP over 5 sec

Side effects

Bleeding, allergic reaction, reperfusion arrhythmias

Considerations

- Contraindicated if active bleeding, hemorrhagic stroke, intracranial neoplasm, aortic dissection. There are also numerous relative contraindications for physician consideration.
- May be administered with aspirin and/or heparin

Flumazenil

Romazicon

Classification

Benzodiazepine antagonist

Indication

Oversedation or respiratory depression as a result of benzodiazepine administration or ingestion

Dosage

0.2 mg IV over 15 sec, followed by 0.3 mg IV over 30 sec if needed, followed by 0.5 mg IV over 30 sec if needed; may repeat 0.5 mg IV q 1 min up to max total dose 3 mg

Considerations

- Monitor for resedation after administration; effects of many benzodiazepines last longer than effects of reversal agent
- Use caution in seizure-prone patients—benzodiazepines will not be effective once this medication is used

Furosemide

Lasix

Classification

Loop diuretic

Indications

Pulmonary edema

Actions

- Venodilation: causing reduced central venous pressure
- Inhibits the reabsorption of sodium in the kidneys, causing diuresis

Dosage

0.5–1.0 mg/kg over 1–2 min (generally given in 20 mg increments)

Route

IV push slowly

Side effects

- Dehydration
- Tinnitus
- Hypokalemia

Glycoprotein IIb/IIIa Inhibitors

Indications

- Chest pain with ST segment depression
- NSTEMI
- Unstable angina
- Patients undergoing percutaneous cardiac intervention

Action

Blocks enzyme glycoprotein IIb/IIIa, which is essential for platelet aggregation

Dosage

- *Eptifabide* (Integrilin): 180 mcg/kg IVP over 1–2 min followed by infusion of 2 mcg/min (decrease to 0.5 mcg/min precardiac cath). Drug available in 100 ml bolus vials and 100 ml infusion vials, which can be spiked directly for administration.
- *Tirofiban* (Aggrastat): Infuse 0.4 mcg/kg/min × 30 min and then 0.1 mcg/kg/min in combination with heparin for 48–108 hr
- *Abciximab* (ReoPro): 0.25 mg/kg IVP followed by infusion of 10 mcg/min

Considerations

- Side effects: bleeding (more likely in females, patient < 75 lb, > 65 yr, hx of GI disease, or receiving fibrinolytics), nausea, vomiting, hypotension, bradycardia
- Further risk of bleeding when used in combination with aspirin and heparin
- Contraindicated if active bleeding or bleeding past 30 days
- Contraindicated if platelets < 100,000, SBP > 180, DBP > 100

Heparin—Unfractionated

Classification

Anticoagulant

Indications

- Patients undergoing angioplasty
- Selected patients receiving fibrinolytic therapy
- In MI patients for pulmonary embolism prophylaxis until fully ambulatory

Actions

Prevents conversion of fibrinogen to fibrin and prothrombin to thrombin

Dosage

Bolus dose of 60 U/kg followed by infusion of 12 U/kg/hr

Side effects

Hemorrhage, thrombocytopenia

Contraindications

Active bleeding, peptic ulcer disease, severe hepatic disease, hemophilia

Heparin—Fractionated Low Molecular Weight Heparin

Enoxaparin (Lovenox, Clexane), Dalteparin (Fragmin)

Classification

Anticoagulant

Indications

- Chest pain with ST depression or positive cardiac markers
- Unstable angina
- NSTEMI

Actions

Inhibits clotting factor X; only slightly affects thrombin, PT, and PTT

Dosage

- *Enoxaparin* (Lovenox): 1 mg/kg sq q 12 hrs in conjunction with aspirin (no IM or IV). Give for minimum of 2 days.
- *Dalteparin* (Fragmin): 120 U/kg sq q 12 hr × 5–8 days

Adverse reactions

- Bleeding, ecchymosis
- Spinal column hematomas in patients post spinal or epidural anesthesia

Contraindications

- Sensitivity to heparin or pork products
- Caution in patients with heparin-induced thrombocytopenia, renal insufficiency, or who are elderly

Lidocaine

Xylocaine

Classification

Antiarrhythmic

Indications

VF, VT, PVCs

Actions

- Depresses ventricular irritability and automaticity
- Increases fibrillation threshold

Dosage

- PVCs, stable VT: 0.5–0.75 mg/kg, may repeat q 5–10 min to max total dose 3 mg/kg
- VF and VT: 1–1.5mg/kgm, may repeat at ½ dose q 5-10 min, to max 3 mg/kg
- Maintenance infusion: 2 gm/500 cc D5W = 4 mg/cc; infuse at 1–4 mg/min (15–60 cc/hr)

Route

IV/IO, ET, IV infusion

Considerations

- Monitor for signs of toxicity: Muscle tremors, paresthesias, CNS symptoms/seizures
- Reduce infusion rate in patients with hepatic dysfunction or left ventricular dysfunction

Quick Tip

Don't give antiarrhythmic drug to bradycardic patients. Premature beats still deliver blood. Remember to stabilize rate, then rhythm, then blood pressure.

Magnesium Sulfate

Classification

Antiarrhythmic (electrolyte)

Indications

- Refractory ventricular arrhythmias
- Torsades de pointes
- Life-threatening arrhythmias due to digitalis toxicity
- Hypomagnesemia

Actions

Stabilizes tissue membranes (including myocardial cells), elevates magnesium levels

Dosage

- VF: 1–2 gm IV/IO
- VT: 1–2 gm diluted in 10 cc over 1–2 min
- Infusion: 0.5–1.0 gm/hr infusion

Route

IV/IO, IV infusion

Side effects

- Mild bradycardia, hypotension
- Overdose: diarrhea, circulatory collapse, paralysis

Morphine

Classification

Narcotic analgesic

Indications

- Ischemic chest pain
- Pulmonary edema
- Severe pain

Actions

- Potent analgesic
- Promotes venous pooling causing a decrease in preload
- Reduces anxiety

Dosage

2–4 mg increments q 5–15 min until chest pain is relieved

Route

IV/IO slowly

Considerations

- May cause respiratory depression
- Hypotension may occur in hypovolemic patients
- Nausea may occur

Naloxone Hydrochloride

Narcan

Classification

Reversal agent.
Opiate antagonist

Indications

- Respiratory depression due to opiate administration or ingestion

Dosage

- 0.4–2 mg IV/IO, titrating to adequate respiratory rate and effort
- May administer up to 6–10 mg over 10 min

Considerations

- May precipitate withdrawal in opiate addicted patients
- Monitor patient for resedation and respiratory depression; duration of drug is shorter than duration of opiates
- May be given via endotracheal tube if IV/IO not available

Nitroglycerine

Nitrostat, Tridil

Classification

Antianginal; antihypertensive

Indications

- Ischemic chest pain
- AMI with CHF, anterior wall MI (IV use)
- Recurrent angina
- Hypertensive emergency with ACS

Actions

- Smooth muscle dilator causing a decrease in preload, afterload, and a resulting increase in venous pooling, thus reducing the workload of the myocardium
- May also reduce coronary artery vasospasm

Dosage

- Tablet or metered spray: 1 sl (0.3–0.4 mg dose) q 5 min not to exceed 3
- Infusion: 10–20 μg/min (Mix 50 mg/250 cc = 200 μg/cc. Start at approximately 3 cc/hr and titrate.)
- If sublingual not available, IV bolus 12.5–25 μg followed by infusion

Considerations

- Caution in right ventricular infarction
- May cause hypotension due to venodilation
- Contraindicated in severe bradycardia (<50 bpm) or tachycardia (>110 bpm)
- Contraindicated in presence of phosphodiesterase inhibitor erectile dysfunction drug use
- Contraindicated if SBP < 90

Nitroprusside

Nipride

Classification

Antianginal, antihypertensive

Indications

- Hypertension
- CHF with pulmonary edema
- To decrease afterload in acute mitral or aortic valve regurgitation

Actions

Smooth muscle dilator causing a decrease in preload, afterload, and a resulting increase in venous pooling

Dosage

Infusion: Mix 50 mg/250 cc D5W (200 μg/cc) and start at 0.5–8.0 μg/kg/min

Considerations

- May cause hypotension
- May cause headaches, nausea, vomiting, abdominal cramping
- Should be administered via infusion pump
- Ideally, monitor blood pressure via invasive lines
- Light-sensitive solution; cover IV bag and tubing
- Thiocyanate toxicity possible in patients unable to excrete metabolites

Norepinephrine

Levophed

Classification

Adrenergic stimulator (sympathetic nervous system). Vasopressor

Indications

- Hypotension, SBP <70 mm Hg with low systemic vascular resistance
- Hypotension refractory to Dopamine

Actions

Primarily alpha effects causing an increase in systemic vascular resistance through vasoconstriction

Dosage

Mix 4 mg/250 cc D5W or NS-16 μg/cc. Begin infusion at 0.5–1.0 μg/min (2–4 cc/hr) and titrate to desired BP, up to 30 μg/min (average adult dose is 2–12 μg/min).

Considerations

- Increases myocardial oxygen demand, since the heart must pump against increased resistance. Monitor for signs of myocardial ischemia.
- May cause arrhythmias. Maintain EKG monitoring.
- Extravasation causes tissue necrosis. Infiltrate extravasation area with phentolamine solution.

Oxygen

Indications

- All patients with acute chest pain that may be due to cardiac ischemia
- Suspected hypoxia of any cause
- Cardiac arrest
- Suspected stroke

Actions

Reverses hypoxia

Dosage

Breathing patient:

Nasal cannula @ 1–6 lpm = 21–44% FiO_2

Simple plastic face mask @ 6–10 lpm = 40–60% FiO_2

Non-rebreather mask @ 6–15 lpm = 60–100% FiO_2

Patient with inadequate rate or depth of respirations:

Bag valve mask @ 10–15 lpm with an oxygen reservoir = 90–100% FiO_2

Considerations

- Rare complications in patients with hypoxic respiratory drive. *Never* withhold O_2.

Quick Tip

Let the Patient's Need Be Your Guide

In general:

- Administer low-flow oxygen for patients with chest pain or stroke.
- Ventilate 8–10 breaths per minute for the apneic patient.
- Deliver just enough volume to see the chest rise, around 500–600 cc.

Procainamide

Classification

Antiarrhythmic

Indications

- Pharmacological conversion of supraventricular arrhythmias (especially atrial fibrillation and atrial flutter) to sinus rhythm
- Control of rapid ventricular rate due to accessory pathway in atrial fibrillation with Wolff-Parkinson-White syndrome
- Stable VT or wide complex tachycardias that cannot be distinguished as being supraventricular or ventricular

Actions

- Depresses atrial and ventricular automaticity
- Slows down conduction through all the pacemakers

Dosage

- 20–50 mg/min infusion (1 gm/50 cc @ 60–150 cc/hr) not to exceed 17 mg/kg
- Maintenance infusion: Mix 2 gm/500 cc D5W (= 4 mg/cc). Infuse @ 1–4 mg/min (15–60 cc/hr)

Considerations

- Hypotension may occur (especially with rapid injection)
- Stop administration if widening of qRs complex to >50% of baseline occurs
- Avoid use in patients with preexisting prolonged QT interval and Torsades de pointes
- May have proarrhythmic effects, especially in setting of hypokalemia, hypomagnesemia, AMI

Sodium Bicarbonate

$NaHCO_3$

Classification

Alkalinizer, buffer

Indications

- Metabolic acidosis from any cause (arrest, shock, renal failure, ketoacidosis)
- Tricyclic antidepressant overdose
- Hyperkalemia

Actions

Increases pH, reverses acidosis

Dosage

1 mEq/kg IV push, followed by 0.5 mEq/kg q 10 min based on ABGs (may be given as a slow infusion in overdosed patients where bicarb is indicated)

Considerations

- Not appropriate for respiratory acidosis
- Ensure that IV line is flushed well before and after medication administration

Quick Tip

The "Give one amp of bicarb" routine works only on TV. Unless the patient weighs 50 kg, one amp is underdosing. Pay attention to weight-based dosing.

Vasopressin

Classification

Naturally occurring antidiuretic hormone, nonadrenergic peripheral vasoconstrictor

Indications

An alternative to the first or second dose of epinephrine in all cardiac arrest:
Ventricular fibrillation/pulseless ventricular tachycardia
Pulseless electrical activity
Asystole

Actions

- Causes vasoconstriction by direct stimulation of smooth muscle V1 receptors
- No increase in myocardial oxygen demand
- Increases coronary perfusion pressures, vital organ blood flow, and cerebral oxygen delivery during CPR

Dosage

40 U IV/IO one time

Route

IV push

Adverse effects

Tachycardia, hypertension, PVCs

Verapamil

Isoptin, Calan

Classification

Antiarrhythmic (calcium channel antagonist)

Indications

Supraventricular tachyarrhythmias

Actions

- Calcium channel antagonist
- Slows conduction
- Smooth muscle dilation

Dosage

- 2.5–5 mg IVP over 1–2 min
- May repeat at 5–10 mg after 15–30 min *or* administer 5 mg IV/IO q 15 min to total of 30 mg

Route

IV push slowly

Side effects

Bradycardia, hypotension (do not use in patient with WPW history)

Practice Test Pharmacology Overview

1. Indications

Match the following medications with indications for their use in ACLS:

______ 1. Adenosine

______ 2. Amiodarone

______ 3. Aspirin

______ 4. Atropine sulfate

______ 5. Beta blockers

______ 6. Calcium chloride

______ 7. Diltiazem

______ 8. Dopamine

______ 9. Epinephrine

______ 10. Fibrinolytics

______ 11. Heparin

______ 12. Lidocaine

______ 13. Magnesium sulfate

______ 14. Morphine sulfate

______ 15. Nitroglycerine

______ 16. Norepinephrine

______ 17. Oxygen

______ 18. Procainamide

______ 19. Sodium Bicarbonate

______ 20. Vasopressin

A. Suspected MI, unstable angina

B. Cardiac arrest and symptomatic bradycardia refractory to atropine, pacing, and dopamine

C. AMI with ST elevation in two related leads, with symptoms <12 hours

D. Refractory VF, torsades de pointes

E. Acute coronary syndromes; anyone with chest pain symptoms

F. Recurrent or intermittent VT, VF, SVT

G. Stable reentry SVT

H. Stable VT, or VF/pulseless VT

I. Chest pain or CHF

J. Hyperkalemia or calcium channel blocker overdose

K. Cardiac arrest, arrhythmias, suspected hypoxia, AMI, stroke

L. Stable VT, Useful in the presence of impaired left Ventricular function, VF/pulseless VT, SVT

M. Pressor agent in cardiac arrest, alternative to epinephrine in VF

N. Acute coronary syndrome chest pain unrelieved by Nitroglycerin. Pulmonary edema without hypotension

O. Hyperkalemia, metabolic acidosis

P. Refractory PSVT, or rapid atrial fibrillation or flutter

Q. SBP <70 mm Hg

R. AMI when fibrinolytics administered

S. Symptomatic sinus bradycardia

T. SBP 70–100 mm Hg and no signs of shock

2. Doses

Write the correct dose for the drug/diagnosis described.

______ 21. Atropine for symptomatic bradycardia

______ 22. Adenosine for stable SVT

______ 23. Vasopressin for VF

______ 24. Lidocaine for stable VT

_______25. Oxygen for bradycardia without repiratory distress

_______26. Amiodarone for VF

_______27. Epinephrine for asystole

_______28. Sodium bicarbonate

_______29. Maximum total dose of Atropine

_______30. Procainamide for VT

_______31. Aspirin for chest pain

_______32. Lidocaine infusion

_______33. Amiodarone for stable VT

_______34. Maximum total dose of Lidocaine

_______35. Morphine for chest pain of pulmonary edema

_______36. Atropine for PEA with heart rate 55/min

_______37. Nitroglycerine sl for chest pain

_______38. Oxygen via BVM in cardiorespiratory arrest

_______39. Dopamine infusion for hypotension

_______40. Epinephrine via ET for VF

41. Your patient is experiencing chest pain, has been placed on oxygen, the ECG monitor, and given 2 aspirin. His blood pressure is 150/94, heart rate is 108, respirations 18, O_2 saturation 98% and ECG reveals sinus tachycardia with occasional PVCs. You are planning to establish venous access on this patient. Which is most appropriate based on his condition?
    A. An 18 ga catheter in the external jugular.
    B. A 20 ga catheter in the forearm.
    C. An intraosseous catheter before he arrests.
    D. This patient does not require an IV at this time.

42. Which of the following vascular access sites poses the greatest risk of complications?
    A. An intraosseous placed in the tibia.
    B. A 16 ga catheter in the external jugular.
    C. A subclavian line placed by the physician.
    D. A 20 ga catheter in the dorsum of the foot.

43. During cardiac arrest which of the following vascular access points is most appropriate?
    A. Internal jugular as the first "IV" attempt.
    B. 16 ga catheter in the saphenous vein.
    C. Sternal intraosseous as the first "IV" attempt.
    D. 18 gauge in the antecubital fossa.

44. You are managing a 60-year-old male who has just converted from ventricular fibrillation to asystole. Epinephrine was administered via a peripheral IV site. If the patient fails to respond to this first medication, when should the next medication be administered?

    A. In 1–2 minutes.

    B. Immediately.

    C. 5–10 minutes later.

    D. In 5 minutes.

45. In a patient who is being managed during cardiac arrest, which of the following should be accomplished each time a medication is administered through a peripheral IV site?

    A. Elevate the extremity the medication was pushed in.

    B. Perform CPR for 2 minutes to circulate the medication.

    C. Flush 20 ml of IV fluid through the IV following the medication.

    D. All of the above.

CHAPTER

7 Stroke

Stroke: What Is It?

The term *stroke* (formerly CVA, or cerebrovascular accident) is used to describe the development of neurologic symptoms caused by brain ischemia or hemorrhage. Stroke is an emergency, and it is caused by inadequate blood flow to brain cells, because vessels feeding that brain tissue have become occluded or have ruptured. Shortly after brain cells are deprived of blood flow, and therefore, oxygen, they begin to die, resulting in the impairment of some of the functions of whatever part of the brain is involved. Signs of stroke can include motor weakness or paralysis, difficulty with speech, swallowing or balance, changes in alertness or orientation, or alteration in sensation, perception, or vision.

A similar clinical presentation may occur with TIA (transient ischemic attack), which is due to temporary disruption in circulation to a portion of the brain, causing symptoms that are stroke like, but resolve shortly after they occur. It is impossible to distinguish between the two in the initial presentation.

Risk

Most patients who have a stroke have identifiable risk factors. Some of the risk factors can be altered, such as hypertension (control with medication), smoking (cessation), history of TIAs (anticoagulation therapy), diabetes (good blood sugar control), carotid artery narrowing (endarterectomy if high-grade stenosis). Other risk factors are not modifiable, such as age, gender, past history of stroke, race, or family history of stroke. Patients with identified risk factors, especially ones with some unmodifiable factors, should be counseled to work on any modifiable risks they might have to decrease their risk of stroke.

Two types of stroke exist: *hemorrhagic stroke,* caused by bleeding in the brain, causing disruption of circulation and compression of brain tissue, and *ischemic stroke,* cause by occlusion of a vessel, leading to impaired circulation. The most aggressive treatment for ischemic stroke is fibrinolytic therapy, which breaks ups clots that lodge in cerebral vessels, restoring blood flow. However, since brain cells are very sensitive to low perfusion states, reperfusion via fibrinolytic therapy must be accomplished quickly, within 3 hours of onset of stroke symptoms. Early recognition of strokelike symptoms and early diagnosis of stroke may facilitate early and aggressive treatment, which may restore blood flow to areas of the brain and save that tissue and associated neurologic function.

A sequence of actions and decisions must be activated rapidly if your patient's **DATA** will help him **SCORE** reversal of the stroke symptoms:

D Detect symptoms that brain cells are deprived of circulation.

A Alert EMS or the appropriate caretaker in your facility.

T Transport the patient to the appropriate medical facility, *or,* for inpatients, transport the appropriate people to the patient for evaluation.

A Assess and reassess more thoroughly, focusing on indications or contraindications for fibrinolytic therapy.

S Scan the brain (CT scan) to rule out hemorrhagic infarction.

C Choose treatment after weighing pros and cons.

O Options may include including fibrinolytic therapy, interventional radiology procedures, other pharmaceutical treatment.

R Reperfuse, if appropriate, within 3 hours of onset of symptoms.

E Evaluate patient status and progress during and after fibrinolytic therapy.

Detect

The symptoms that a patient may display as he is having a stroke will vary, depending on which part of the brain is affected. Early in the evolution of the stroke, symptoms may be subtle. The ability of the ACLS provider to detect subtle signs of stroke is critical to early diagnosis and treatment. In addition to detecting stroke symptoms, the ACLS provider should be alert to nonstroke causes of strokelike behavior, such as hypoglycemia and toxicology, and treat those causes if they are the reasons for the patient's deficit. Figure 7-1 shows common signs and symptoms of stroke and TIA.

There are three neurologic signs that, if abnormal, are good predictors that your patient is having a stroke, so be sure to assess for *slurred speech, facial asymmetry*, and *arm drift*.

SLURRED SPEECH

To determine whether patients' speech is slurred, talk to them! Speech difficulties can be due either to difficulties with the speech center in the brain (dysphasia) or weakness in the muscles necessary for speech (dysarthria). Some professionals work with stroke assessment scales that include phrases that you might ask the patient to repeat after you to test their ability to speak. In other settings, specific stroke scales are not used, and the provider merely relies on conversation with the patient to assess the speech. No matter how you assess the patient, be alert for slurring of words, slow speech, difficulty forming words, or problems choosing correct or appropriate words. If speech is not normal, consider that the patient is having a stroke until proven otherwise, and act accordingly.

Figure 7-1 Stroke (cerebrovascular accident or CVA) and transient ischemic attack (TIA) are conditions that may result from nontraumatic brain injury. Loss of speech, sensory, or motor function and altered mental status are among the possible signs and symptoms.

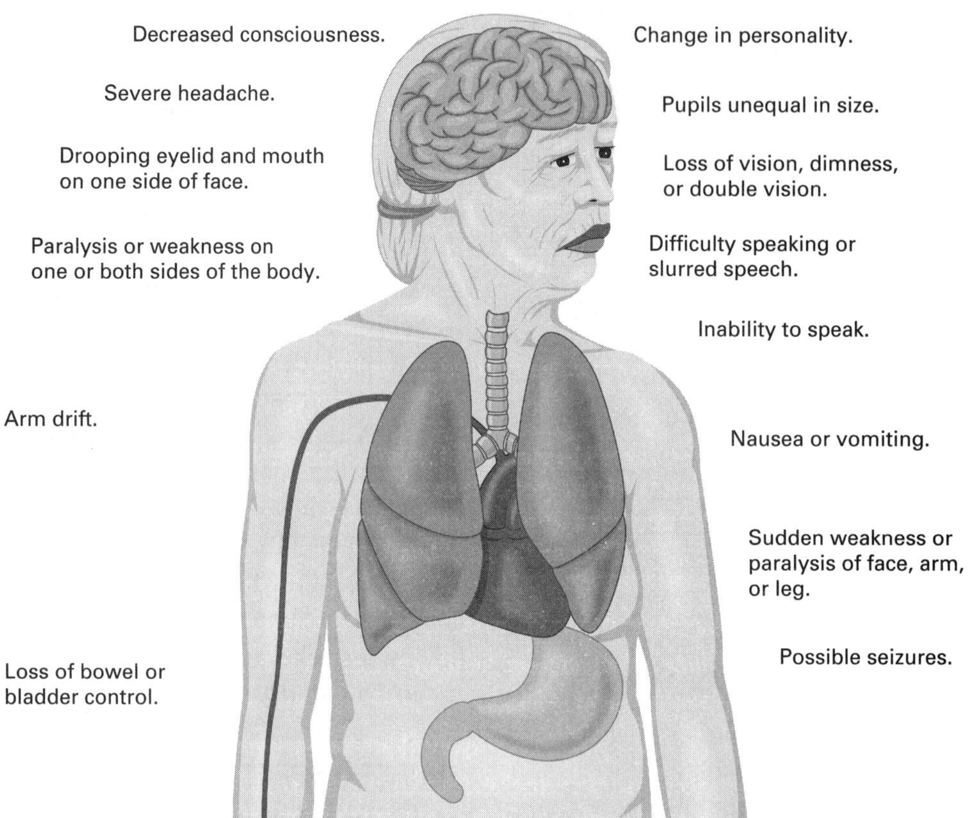

FACIAL ASYMMETRY

A face that is asymmetrical is caused by weakness in the facial muscles and can be caused by stroke. Facial droop can be missed in a face that is at rest, so it is important to ask the patient to move his mouth so you are able to tell whether or not one side is weak. "Please smile" or "Show me your teeth" are two requests that you can make of the patient that will prompt him to try to elevate his lips, revealing asymmetry if it is present (Figure 7-2).

ARM DRIFT

A deficit in upper extremity motor strength can be easily noted if the patient is unable to move or has significant weakness, but is more difficult to detect if weakness is mild. Again, early recognition of stroke symptoms plays a key role in early and effective treatment, so you should assess strength in all patients with possible stroke, even if gross weakness or paralysis is not present. One way to test for upper extremity weakness is to check for arm drift. Ask your patient to close his eyes, and extend his arms in front of him, palms up, and maintain that position. A rotation, drifting, or dropping of one of those arms indicates weakness that should be noted and considered to be due to stroke until proven otherwise (Figure 7-3).

Figure 7-2a The face of a nonstroke patient has normal symmetry.

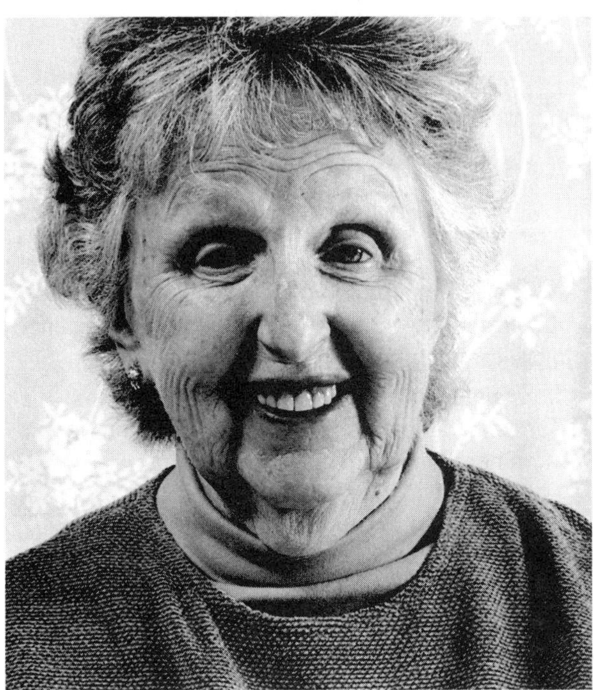

Figure 7-3a The patient who has not suffered a stroke can generally hold arms in an extended position with eyes closed.

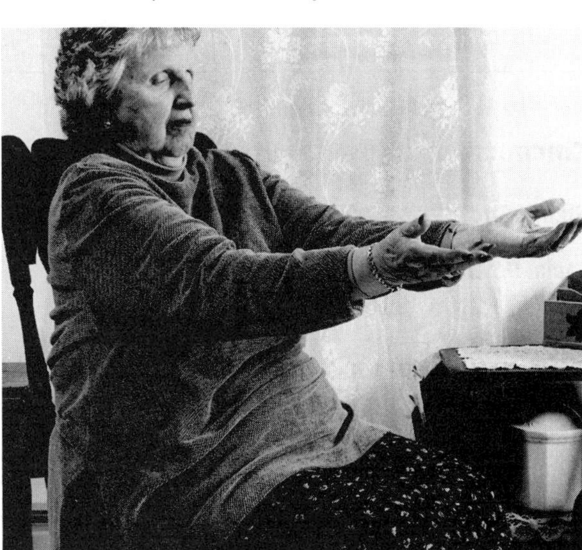

Figure 7-2b The face of a stroke patient often has an abnormal, drooped appearance on one side.

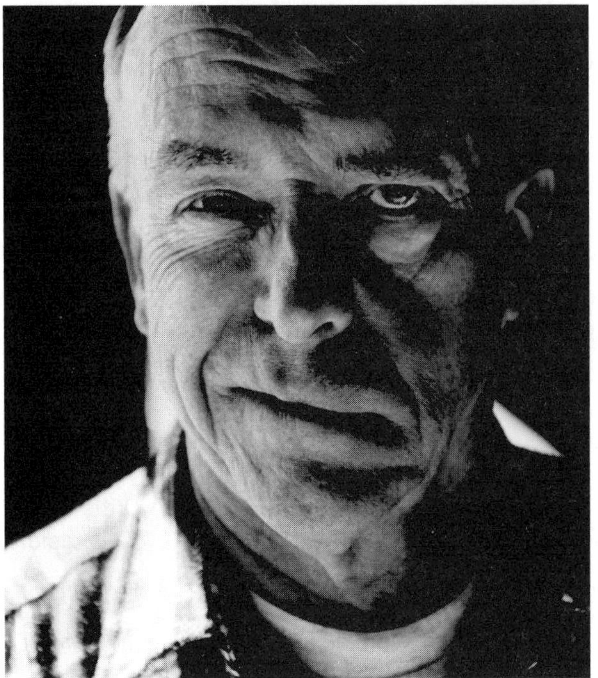

Figure 7-3b A stroke patient will often display "arm drift" or "pronater drift"; that is, one arm will remain extended, when held outward with eyes closed, but the other arm will drift or drop downward and pronate (turn palm downward).

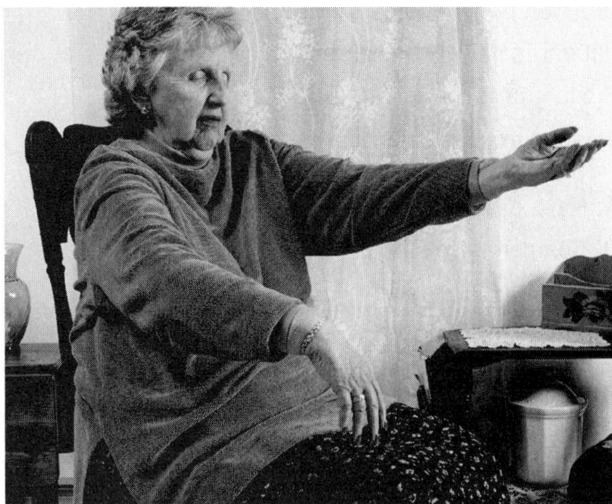

The Cincinnati Prehospital Stroke Scale (Figure 7-4) and the Los Angeles Prehospital Stroke Screen (LAPSS) (Figure 7-5) are among the screening tools that providers can use to detect and document neurologic deficit that may be stroke related.

Figure 7-4 The Cincinnati Prehospital Stroke Scale

Cincinnati Prehospital Stroke Scale

Sign of Stroke	Patient Activity	Interpretation
Facial Droop	Have patient look up at you, smile, and show his teeth.	*Normal:* Symmetry to both sides. *Abnormal:* One side of the face droops or does not move symmetrically.
Arm Drift	Have patient lift arms up and hold them out with eyes closed for ten seconds.	*Normal:* Symmetrical movement in both arms. *Abnormal:* One arm drifts down or asymmetrical movement of the arms.
Abnormal Speech	Have the patient say "you can't teach an old dog new tricks."	*Normal:* The correct words are used and no slurring of words is noted. *Abnormal:* The words are slurred, the wrong words are used, or the patient is aphasic.

Kothari RU, Pancioli A, Liu T, Broderick J. Cincinnati Prehospital Stroke Scale: reproducibility and validity. Annals of Emergency Medicine. *1999;33:373–378.*

Figure 7-5 The Los Angeles Prehospital Stroke Screen

Los Angeles Prehospital Stroke Screen (LAPSS)

Considerations	Yes	Unknown	No
Age **greater than** 45 years			
No history of seizures or epilepsy			
Duration of symptoms is **less** than 24 hours			
Patient is **not** wheelchair bound or bedridden			
Blood glucose level **between 60 and 400 mg/dl**			
Physical exam to determine unilateral asymmetry	**Equal**	**R Weakness**	**L Weakness**
A. Have patient look up, smile, and show teeth		Droop	Droop
B. Compare grip strength of upper extremities		Weak grip No grip	Weak grip No grip
C. Assess arm strength for drift or weakness		Drifts down Falls rapidly	Drifts down Falls rapidly

Kidwell CS, Saver JL, Schubert GB, Eckstein M, Starkman S. Design and retrospective analysis of the Los Angeles Prehospital Stroke Screen (LAPSS). Prehospital Emergency Care. *1998;2:267–273.*
Kidwell CS, Starkman S, Eckstein M, Weems K, Saver JL. Identifying stroke in the field: prospective validation of the Los Angeles Prehospital Stroke Screen (LAPSS). Stroke. *2000;31:71–76.*

Alert

Further assessment, diagnosis, and treatment can occur only if the appropriate individuals are alerted of the patient's problem. This means calling 911 for patients outside of the healthcare setting, and notifying the appropriate caregivers and diagnostic departments for patients already in a hospital bed.

Transport

For patients in the prehospital setting, rapid screening at the scene (often including one of the aforementioned stroke screening tools), ruling out nonstroke causes of any deficits, support of vital functions (ABCs), and rapid transport to a facility equipped to diagnose and treat stroke patients rapidly should occur. Time should not be wasted on scene for any other interventions (IV, for example, which can be started en route).

For the hospitalized patient, people and services necessary to further evaluate the patient's status should go to the patient, without delay. Give indications for treatment, and rule out nonstroke causes of the deficit.

Quick Tip

Time is brain! The priority with the patient exhibiting stroke symptoms is to stabilize and determine eligibility for fibrinolytic therapy. This means ruling out nonstroke causes of the deficit, determining time of onset of the symptoms, and ruling out hemorrhage with a CT scan.

Assess

A targeted history and more thorough exam should take place. One goal of the in-depth phase of data gathering is to determine the appropriateness and safety of administration of fibrinolytic drugs. Important information to obtain includes the following:

- Time of onset of the symptoms. If the patient is not sure, ask family members or whoever was with the patient at the time. This is a critical piece of information, necessary when making the decision regarding use of fibrinolytic drugs. Administration of fibrinolytic therapy is contraindicated after 3 hours following onset of symptoms.
- What was the patient doing when the symptoms began? It is important to rule out any type of trauma that may have caused a head injury, causing a neuro deficit. Try to distinguish between the patient who fell, hit his head, then experienced weakness or other deficit, from the patient who experienced weakness in a lower extremity and then fell.
- What other symptoms does the patient have? Symptoms such as seizures, stiff neck, and severe headache are often present when the stroke is hemorrhagic in origin. Fibrinolytic therapy is absolutely contraindicated in hemorrhagic stroke.
- Are there any other findings that would be factors in the decision to use or not use fibrinolytic therapy, such as:
  - Is there hypertension that does not respond to medication?
  - Does the patient have a history of previous stroke?
  - Is the patient on anticoagulant therapy?
  - Have the symptoms gotten better since they began?

Scan

The patient should very rapidly be sent for a noncontrast CT scan to rule out hemorrhagic stroke. A CT scan that is positive for acute stroke indicates hemorrhage and is a contraindication for fibrinolytic therapy. A scan that is normal indicates absence of hemorrhage but does not rule out stroke. The changes caused by ischemic strokes are not detected by CT scan until a few days after the initial event. The CT scan personnel should be notified as soon as the stroke is suspected, so the stroke patient's scan is not delayed by other patient's tests.

Choose

Based on CT results, a therapy must be chosen.

Options

Treatment options include:

- Fibrinolytic therapy—for patients with ischemic stroke, symptoms that began less than 3 hours ago, with no other contraindications
- Clot retrieval procedures—for patients with ischemic stroke, in settings where neuroradiology services are available
- Surgery—for patients with hemorrhagic stroke that causes compression of structures and is surgically accessible, or to repair vascular defects that caused hemorrhage
- Supportive care, including monitoring and maintaining ABCs, blood pressure control, and early physical, occupational, and speech therapy

Reperfuse

Oxygenated blood must get to brain tissue before cells die. If fibrinolytic therapy is chosen, it must be begun quickly, within 3 hours of onset of the symptoms. Refer to your hospital formulary for details on administration of the particular agent ordered for this patient.

Evaluate

Frequently evaluate the patient's status during and after fibrinolytic therapy. Watch for, report, and document improvement of symptoms (which may indicate successful restoration of circulation to the ischemic area of brain) or worsening of symptoms (which may indicate hemorrhage in the brain). Even with successful therapy, the patient's symptoms may not resolve right away, but may gradually improve in the coming days and weeks.

Practice Test 1 Stroke

Your 80-year-old neighbor, Mary, tells you about a friend who recently had a stroke. She states, "It's really sad. My friend woke up feeling fine, and a few hours later, she was paralyzed on one side and couldn't talk. I guess there's nothing you can do about a stroke once it hits you."

1. Based on what you know about stroke diagnosis and treatment, you should tell her which of the following:
   A. Once stroke symptoms start, there is nothing that can be done about them, so stroke prevention is key.
   B. If you notice stroke symptoms, either in yourself or someone else, you should call your doctor for further instructions.
   C. Some strokes can be successfully treated if caught early, so anyone noticing stroke symptoms should call 911 immediately.
   D. EMS personnel (paramedics) can administer medications to stop the progression of stroke before the patient even gets to the hospital, so calling 911 is critical when stroke symptoms appear.

2. When Mary tells you to list some common signs of stroke, you should tell her about:
   A. Confusion or other changes in mental status or personality.
   B. Pain when walking.
   C. Weakness or sensory changes on one side of the body.
   D. Difficulty speaking or swallowing.
   E. A, C, and D
   F. B, C, and D

You also talk to Mary about risk factors for stroke, including hypertension, smoking, diabetes, age, gender, and history of stroke.

3. Which of the following is a modifiable risk factor for stroke?
   A. History of prior stroke.
   B. Heredity.
   C. Hypertension.
   D. Race.

4. Mary has multiple medical problems, including glaucoma, diabetes, and a history of unstable angina. This morning at breakfast time, she begins to feel dizzy, and drops her coffee cup because her right hand is weak and numb. Because of what you have told her about stroke symptoms, she calls 911 immediately. The paramedics arrive promptly and conduct their initial assessment and gather history. Which of the following questions is aimed at trying to determine Mary's eligibility for fibrinolytic therapy?
   A. "Did you take your medication this morning?"
   B. "What time did these symptoms begin?"
   C. "What time did you last eat?"
   D. "Are you having any chest pain?"

5. You would expect the paramedics to assess which of the following to rule out nonstroke causes of her dizziness and weakness:
   A. Last time she administered her eyedrops.
   B. Blood pressure.
   C. Blood glucose.
   D. Oxygen saturation.

Mary's blood pressure is 150/90, her heart rate is 98 per minute, her respiratory rate is 18 per minute. Her skin is warm and dry, and her SpO_2 *is 98%. She states that she took all her regular medications this morning, before breakfast. She was eating a muffin and drinking coffee about 20 minutes earlier when her hand became weak and she felt dizzy. She was sitting in a chair and did not fall, but was able to reach the telephone and call 911. She does not have a headache, any chest pain, or difficulty breathing. Her symptoms have not improved since she called the paramedics.*

6. What is the most appropriate next action for the paramedics?
   A. Quickly prepare the patient for transport, alerting the receiving facility that they are transporting a patient with stroke symptoms.
   B. Perform a secondary assessment, with more detailed history and physical.
   C. Establish a peripheral IV and prepare for potential airway or hemodynamic emergency.
   D. Administer oxygen, establish IV, and administer a beta blocker for her hypertension.

7. During transport, the paramedics reassess Mary's neurologic status, being alert for improvement or worsening of her deficits. What is the significance of improving neurologic status?
   A. Early improvement of neuro deficits suggests that Mary would respond favorably to fibrinolytic therapy and make her a good candidate.
   B. Early improvement of neuro status suggests that the cause of the stroke is hemorrhage, making fibrinolytic therapy a contraindication.
   C. Early improvement in neuro status suggests that the cause of the deficit was more likely hypoglycemia or hypoxia, so fibrinolytic therapy is not indicated.
   D. Early improvement of neuro status suggests that the cause of the deficit was more likely TIA, which will continue to resolve, so fibrinolytic therapy is not indicated.

8. Upon arrival to the hospital, which of the following diagnostic tests should be performed as soon as possible?
   A. CT scan of the brain, with IV contrast.
   B. Lumbar puncture, to detect blood in the spinal fluid.
   C. CT scan of the brain without IV contrast.
   D. Lab draw for CBC, electrolytes, and coagulation.

When she arrives in the ED, Mary's blood is drawn, a 2-lead ECG is performed, staff reassesses her neuro status, and she is sent for a CT scan. The physician soon tells Mary and her family that her CT scan is normal.

9. What does a finding of "normal CT" mean in terms of possible treatment?
   A. Mary did not have a stroke. Her course of treatment will depend on the cause of her deficit.
   B. Mary did not have a hemorrhage and may be a candidate for fibrinolytic therapy.
   C. Mary should have an MRI to further evaluate her brain and causes for her deficit.
   D. Mary's stroke is most likely ischemic in nature and she is therefore not a candidate for fibrinolytic therapy.

Patients who are candidates for fibrinolytic therapy must give informed consent prior to administration of the medication. The physician discussed the risks and benefits of fibrinolytic therapy to the patient and family.

10. Which of the following is true about fibrinolytic therapy?
    A. There is potential for intracerebral bleeding in a patient who receives fibrinolytic medications, resulting in tragic outcomes.
    B. There is potential for resolution of stroke symptoms if the occluded vessel in the brain is opened and cells receive adequate circulation before too much damage is done.
    C. Bleeding in areas of the body, other than the brain, can occur following administration of fibrinolytic medications, sometimes with serious or fatal consequences.
    D. There is a possibility that the stroke symptoms may not get worse or better following administration of fibrinolytic medications.
    E. All of the above

Practice Test 2 Stroke

1. Statistics state that less than 10% of patients with acute ischemic stroke are eligible for fibrinolytic therapy. Which of the following best describes the low utilization of this therapy?
   A. Patients decline consent for the treatment after learning the risks and benefits.
   B. Hospital or emergency personnel are often not informed of stroke symptoms soon enough for the patient to receive fibrinolytics within the prescribed time frame.
   C. Few healthcare organizations possess the diagnostic capabilities to rapidly rule out hemorrhagic infarct and determine fibrinolytic eligibility.
   D. Most healthcare providers mistakenly believe that once stroke symptoms begin, they cannot be reversed, and therefore fail to respond quickly to changes in neurologic status.

2. Which of the following is the best course of action if a patient or family member notices sudden onset of speech or vision difficulty, weakness, or dizziness?
   A. Contact the patient's primary physician to see if he is available for an office visit.
   B. Note the time of onset of symptoms and call 911 if symptoms do not resolve in 30 minutes.
   C. Gather a list of the patient's medications and immediately get a ride to the nearest emergency department.
   D. Note the time of onset of symptoms and call 911.

3. Which of the following factors contribute to the delay in diagnosis and treatment of acute ischemic stroke?
   A. Patient being transported to the hospital by family or friends.
   B. Stroke signs that are subtle and difficult to detect.
   C. The expense of stroke care in large urban medical center.
   D. Patient's denial or rationalization of stroke symptoms.
   E. A, B, and C
   F. A, B, and D
   G. B, C, and D

4. Which of the following findings can mimic an acute stroke?
   A. Hyperglycemia.
   B. Acute myoclonic seizures.
   C. Hypokalemia.
   D. Hypoglycemia.

5. Which of the following is not a contraindication for the administration of fibrinolytic medication to treat stroke?
   A. No evidence of stroke on initial CT scan.
   B. CT evidence of intracranial hemorrhage.
   C. Blood pressure 190/110 that does not respond to medications.
   D. Abdominal surgery 2 weeks ago.

6. Mrs. Jones, an 80-year-old diabetic woman, notices weakness in her right hand as she is eating breakfast at 8:30 A.M. She remembers speaking to her doctor about signs of stroke and decides to call 911. Upon arrival, the paramedics should:
   A. Assess vital signs, administer oxygen via nasal cannula, obtain a medical history, perform a general neurological screening assessment, obtain information about the time of onset of symptoms, check blood sugar, alert the nearest stroke facility, and transport immediately.
   B. Obtain blood samples and a detailed medical history, consult patient's primary physician for a treatment plan, check blood sugar, and transport if patient's symptoms do not resolve in 30 minutes.
   C. Assess mental status, speech, and motor function, call the patient's daughter to inquire about the patient's previous neurologic status, transport to the nearest medical facility for evaluation of diabetic complications.
   D. Assess ABCs, administer oxygen via nasal cannula, assess vital signs and perform a general neurologic screening, assess time of onset of symptoms, check blood sugar, and administer IV fibrinolytic medication on scene if there are no noted contraindications.

7. You are watching television with your 75-year-old neighbor. You glance over and see that she is leaning to one side. When you ask if she is okay, she replies with slow, slurred speech. You ask if she takes any medications, and she slowly says "only

vitamins." Which of the following is the most appropriate action for you to take at this time?

A. Call your neighbor's husband and ask him to take her to the hospital.
B. Call 911 and tell the dispatcher that you are with someone who has signs of a stroke.
C. Continue talking with your neighbor for the next few minutes to see if the symptoms resolve.
D. Offer to drive your neighbor to the nearby hospital that just received stroke center status.

8. Following neurologic exam and CT of the brain, the following patients have been diagnosed as having acute ischemic stroke. Which patient has no stated contraindications to fibrinolytic therapy?

A. The 50-year-old woman who noticed weakness on the left side of her mouth 2 hours ago.
B. The 75-year-old woman who was diagnosed with bleeding duodenal ulcers yesterday.
C. The 65-year-old man who woke up 2 hours ago with weakness on the left side of his body.
D. The 50-year-old who is 1-week post radical prostatectomy surgery.

9. A 65-year-old woman is transported to the ED by paramedics who report that they were called to her home for new onset of right-sided weakness, which has worsened since they first assessed her. Her CT scan is reported as negative for hemorrhage. Which of the following is the most important piece of information needed to determine her eligibility for fibrinolytic therapy?

A. Has she had a stroke before?
B. When did the stroke symptoms start?
C. What medications does she take?
D. Is a family member available to sign consent?

10. Which of the following best describes the time frame for administering fibrinolytic medications to the patient with acute ischemic stroke?

A. Fibrinolytic medications must be administered within 3 hours of initial assessment by medical personnel.
B. Fibrinolytic medications must be administered within 30 minutes of arrival at the hospital.
C. Fibrinolytic medications must be administered within 3 hours of the patient waking up with stroke symptoms.
D. Fibrinolytic medications must be administered within 3 hours of onset of stroke symptoms.

CHAPTER

8 Acute Coronary Syndromes

Acute coronary syndromes (ACS) is an umbrella term for situations where perfusion to the myocardium is suboptimal, resulting in clinical symptoms such as chest pain, abnormal laboratory finding such as elevated cardiac markers, or ultimately, infarction, which may cause patient death or long-term complications such as heart failure.

The Progression of Coronary Vessel Occlusion

A continuum of events often leads to significant occlusion of coronary arteries, decreasing perfusion to the myocardium, leading to the development of acute coronary syndromes.

PLAQUE FORMATION

Artherosclerotic plaque form in the coronary arteries of people with genetic predisposition, high- cholesterol diets, and diabetes. This lipid rich structure takes up room in the lumen of the coronary vessel. A narrow vessel may be unable to provide adequate blood flow, causing hypoperfusion and anginal symptoms during times of physical or emotional stress, when myocardial oxygen demand outweighs supply (Figure 8-1).

This plaque may also become unstable and rupture. Plaque rupture is the most common cause of ACS, and occurs when a combination of an inflammatory process in the lining of the vessel and stress from blood flow cause the thin cap of the plaque to rupture. The rupture of the plaque and

Figure 8-1a Early plaque formation

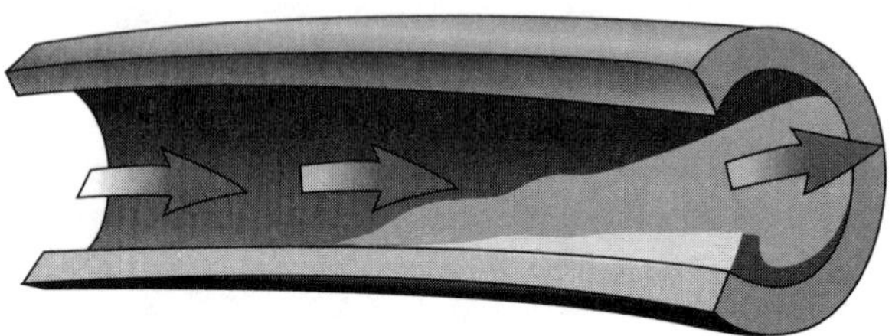

Figure 8-1b Significant plaque formation

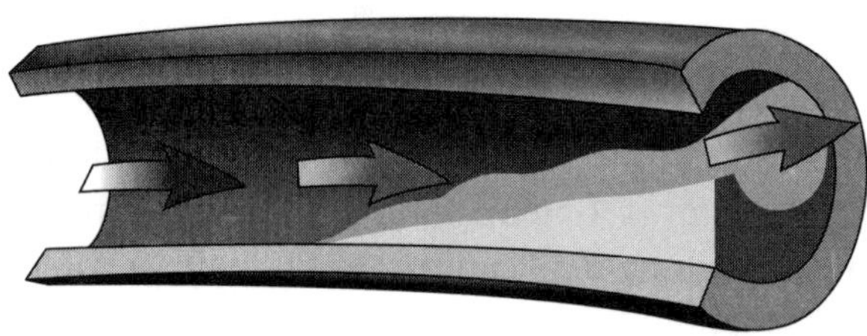

exposure of its contents to the vessel trigger a cascade of events that initially attempt to repair the rupture, but quickly cause some vasoconstriction and form an occlusive clot, impairing blood flow distal to the clot, causing chest pain symptoms.

Plaques that do not rupture still contribute to the development of acute coronary syndromes. Over time, blood cells stick to the wall of the plaque, forming a thrombus, which may partially occlude the lumen of the vessel (Figure 8-2). An occlusive, platelet-rich thrombus may produce ischemia and symptoms, which may even occur when the patient is at rest. Antiplatelet therapy such as Glycoprotein IIb/IIIa inhibitors should be used in these patients to minimize the size of the thrombus and maintain blood flow past the narrowing caused by plaque and thrombus.

Figure 8-2 Significant plaque with partially occlusive clot

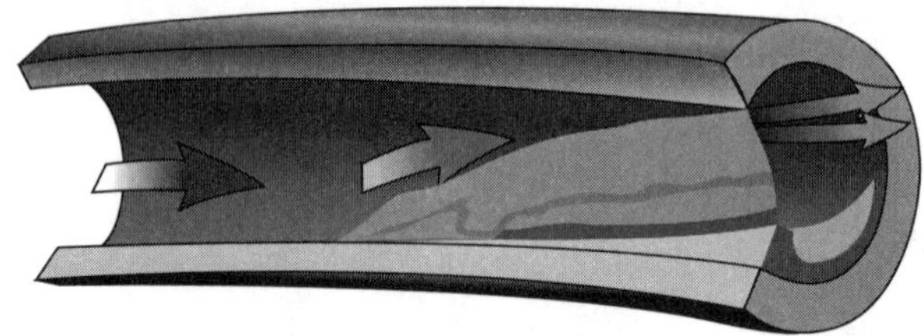

As the thrombus grows larger, small pieces of it may periodically break off, causing small embolic occlusions in the very small distal structures of the coronary arteries.

If the very large clot, now rich in fibrin and thrombin, occludes the vessel, myocardial infarction will occur unless the clot is lysed with fibrinolytic medications or percutaneous intervention (PCI). See Figure 8-3.

LEVELS OF MYOCARDIAL DAMAGE

Lack of oxygen to the myocardium can result in varying levels of myocardial damage, depending on the process involved. Infarction is the end result of evolving changes at the tissue level as a result of oxygen deprivation. We can generalize these three dynamic, overlapping stages as ischemia, injury, and infarction. The earlier the problem is recognized, the sooner the clinician can intervene, and the greater chance there is of preventing infarction or minimizing the size of infarction. See Figure 8-4.

Figure 8-3 Occlusive thrombus

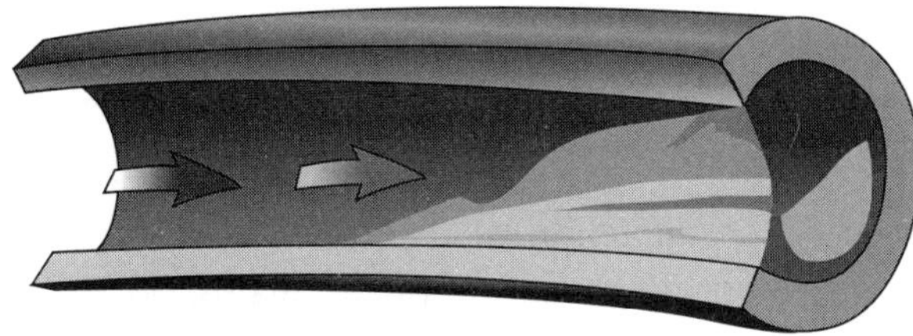

Recognizing a Problem

Selecting the appropriate therapy for a patient experiencing ACS requires that the healthcare provider recognizes the signs of a cardiac emergency early, correctly determines the nature of the emergency, and quickly sets the wheels in motion for therapeutic interventions specific to the patient's problem, with acute myocardial infarction (AMI) being the most serious of all acute coronary syndromes.

Figure 8-4 Stages of AMI

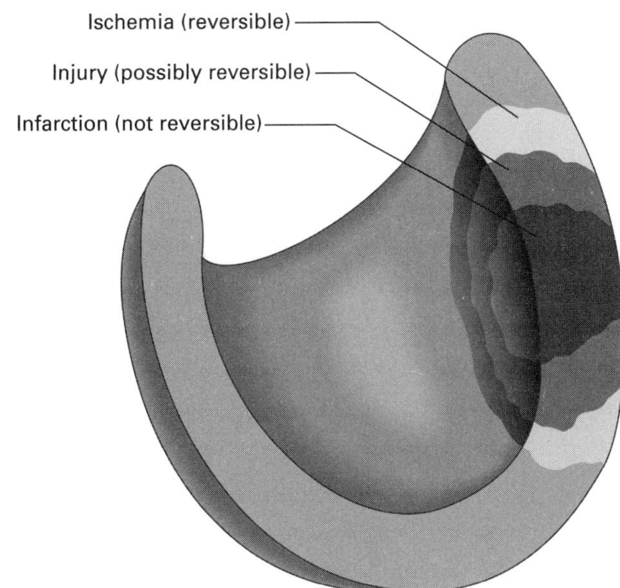

The most common symptom of evolving AMI is chest discomfort that lasts more than a few minutes. The patient may describe it as:

- Chest pain
- Chest pressure
- Squeezing
- Tightness
- Fullness
- Indigestion or heartburn

There may be associated symptoms, such as:

- Pain that spreads to the neck, jaw, back, or shoulders
- General discomfort or anxiety, the feeling that "something is not right"
- Lightheadedness or dizziness
- Diaphoresis
- Nausea
- Shortness of breath

Some patients, including women, diabetics, and elderly patients are less likely to display typical symptoms when experiencing ACS. Be alert to vague complaints in these patients, especially those with clinical history or family history of heart disease.

Some questions that may help you and the patient identify qualities of the pain include:

- "When did the pain begin?"
- "What were you doing when it began?"
- "Is there anything that makes it worse or better?" (positioning, deep breathing)
- "Have you ever had this type of pain before?"
- "On a scale of 0–10 with 0 being no pain and 10 the worst pain you have ever had, can you rate the pain at this time?"

This data will help you and other members of the team distinguish between an AMI and many other imposters (dissecting aneurism, myocarditis, pericarditis, pulmonary embolus, and GI problems, among other things).

Chest pain is often a sign of an oxygen supply-demand mismatch at the level of the myocardium. Initial assessment and treatment is aimed at increasing oxygen supply, while decreasing demand while determining the exact nature of the myocardial problem.

Initial assessment should include:

- Vital signs (T-P-R-BP-O_2 sat)
- Cardiac rhythm (cardiac monitor)
- 12-lead ECG (determine if ischemia, injury, or infarction is occurring)
- Brief targeted history, include criteria for fibrinolytic therapy "just in case"
- Send blood for cardiac markers, coagulation studies, and electrolytes
- Portable chest X ray

Initial treatment should include:

- Establish venous access.
- Administer low-flow oxygen (2–4 lpm) or more if patient's pulmonary status dictates.
- Administer chewable aspirin 162–325 mg.
- Administer sl nitroglycerine, as long as systolic BP > 90.
- Administer morphine sulfate 2–4 mg IV if three doses of nitroglycerine fail to relieve the pain.
- Administer beta blockers to further decrease myocardial oxygen demand.
- Consider using Clopidogrel (Plavix) 300 mg to decrease effectiveness of clot.

As soon as the 12-lead ECG is read, the patient can be placed into one of three groups:

- ST elevation (or new left bundle branch block)
- ST depression or dynamic T-wave inversion
- Normal or nondiagnostic ST and T changes

Each of these categories carries its own specific interventions, as well as implications for possible cardiac emergencies.

PATIENTS WITH ST DEPRESSION (OR DYNAMIC T-WAVE INVERSION)

ST depression $\geq$0.5 mm or T-wave inversion should arouse a strong suspicion for ischemia (see Figures 8-5 and 8-6). There is also a high possibility that the patient is experiencing unstable angina or a non-ST segment elevation MI (NSTEMI). What is critical to remember is that myocardial ischemia is reversible! If the myocardial oxygen supply-demand equation is quickly balanced, no tissue injury will occur.

Unless contraindicated, therapies to decrease myocardial oxygen demand (beta blockers and IV nitroglycerine) and decrease the effectiveness of an occlusive clot, which in turn increases oxygen supply (low-molecular-weight Heparin, aspirin, Clopidogrel, Glycoprotein IIb/IIIa inhibitors), should be implemented. The short-term goal is to equalize the oxygen supply-demand equation and eliminate the chest discomfort. The long-term

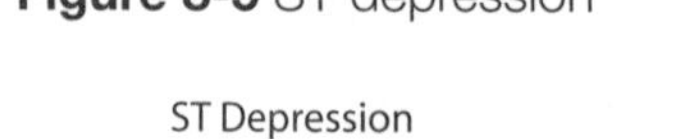
Figure 8-5 ST depression

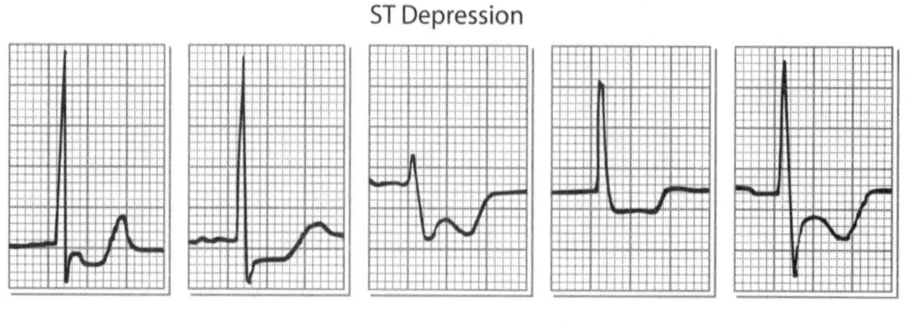

Figure 8-6 T-wave inversion

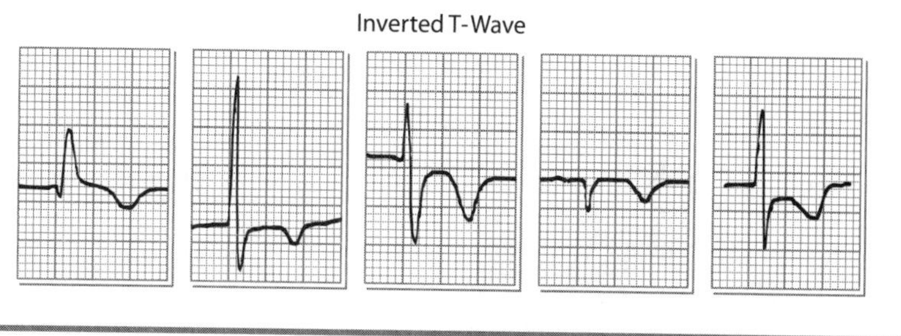

goal is to ensure adequate circulation to the myocardium in the future. If the patient is considered high-risk for infarction or unstable angina, due to any of the following:

- Symptoms not relieved by Morphine, oxygen, Nitroglycerine, aspirin (MONA)
- More than three risk factors for coronary artery disease (CAD)
  - Family history of CAD
  - Diabetes
  - Hypercholesterolemia
  - Hypertension
  - Smoker
- Signs of depressed left ventricular function
- Prior AMI, PCI (Percutaneous Coronary Intervention), or open-heart surgery
- Recurrent ischemia (more than two events in last 24 hours)

then practitioners should perform cardiac catheterization to determine whether there is a stenosis or occlusion that is appropriate for angioplasty, stenting, or bypass grafting. Patients who are lower risk and/or stable may be observed for a longer period of time, with monitoring of serial ECGs and evaluation of cardiac markers. PCI or surgery may still be elected to open severely narrowed coronary vessels. See Figure 8-7.

PATIENTS WITH ST ELEVATION

ST elevation of more than 1 mm in two or more anatomically related leads arouses strong suspicion for myocardial injury (Figure 8-8). Myocardial injury will soon progress to infarction (death of tissue) if oxygenation is not quickly restored to the tissue. This is a class of patients with potential for great benefit from reperfusion therapy, so determining eligibility and quickly implementing reperfusion strategies in these patients is the immediate goal.

REPERFUSION STRATEGIES

Reperfusion strategies may be mechanical (angioplasty, stenting) or chemical (fibrinolytic drugs). The intervention chosen may depend on a number of factors, including resources, time of onset of symptoms, and the presence of other risk factors or contraindications to a particular therapy.

Percutaneous Cardiac Interventions (PCI)

If an interventional cardiac catheterization lab is available, the patient should undergo angioplasty or stenting as soon as possible. A balloon-tipped catheter is introduced into the vascular system through the skin, and threaded into the occluded coronary artery. The balloon is then inflated, opening the vessel. Alternatively, a firm mesh "tube" (stent) is placed at the level of vessel narrowing to keep the vessel open. These interventions should occur shortly after the onset of symptoms, ideally within 90 minutes, to restore circulation to the heart muscle before significant damage occurs.

Fibrinolytic Therapy

If angioplasty or stenting is not available, then fibrinolytic medications may be used to loosen

Figure 8-7 Changes reflecting ischemia, injury, and infarction

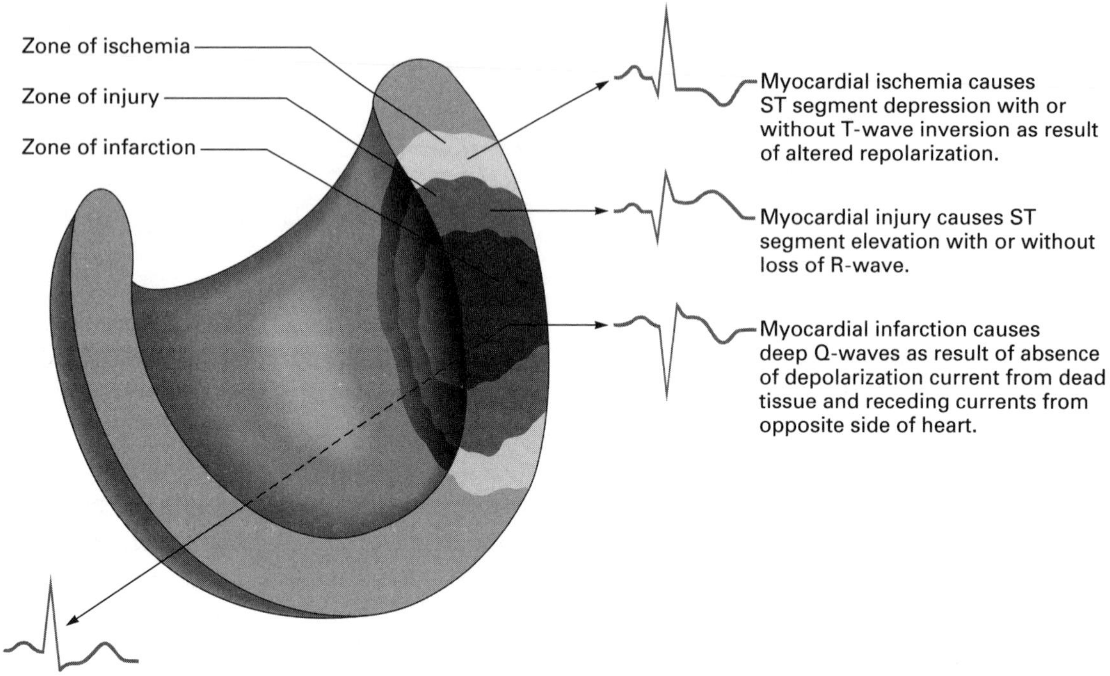

the fibrin net that holds together an occlusive clot, allowing blood flow through and past the clot to the oxygen-deprived myocardium. Ideally, this occurs early after the onset of symptoms and prevents infarction of the tissue.

Since fibrinolytic medications alter the effects of clots, the major unwanted effect is bleeding, particularly bleeding in areas of the body that cannot be compressed. Intracerebral and intraabdominal bleeding can have lethal consequences. Therefore, prior to administering fibrinolytics, practitioners should screen for contraindications of fibrinolytic medications, which include:

- Active internal bleeding within the last 3 weeks
- Known bleeding disorders
- Traumatic injury or major surgery within the last 2 weeks

Figure 8-8 ST elevation

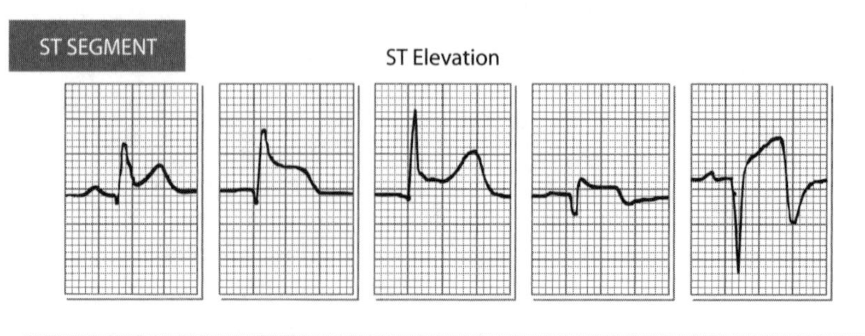

- History of stroke, intracranial neoplasm, aneurism, trauma or surgery to head or spinal column within 3 months
- Uncontrolled hypertension
- Recent lumbar puncture or arterial puncture at a noncompressible site
- Recent CPR with evidence of chest trauma

If any of these exclusion criteria are present, the risks of fibrinolytic therapy significantly outweigh the risks. If fibrinolytic therapy is determined to be appropriate, it should be implemented as soon as possible, ideally within 30 minutes of the time symptoms are reported, and definitely within 12 hours of onset of symptoms.

If more than 12 hours have passed since the onset of chest pain symptoms, it is likely that little heart muscle will be saved by high-risk reperfusion strategies, so fibrinolytics are not indicated, and the appropriateness of an angioplasty procedure may be determined following a diagnostic cardiac catheterization. For this reason, time is of the essence when dealing with patients with symptoms that may be cardiac in nature.

PATIENTS WITH PATHOLOGIC Q-WAVES

If oxygenation is not restored to myocardial cells quickly enough, the tissue will infarct (die). Areas of infarction do not depolarize, and within a few hours can also cause abnormalities on the 12-lead ECG. Pathologic Q-waves are Q-waves (the first downward deflection before the R-wave) that are deeper and wider than the Q-waves found in a normally perfusing heart. The appearance of Q-waves indicates that tissue death has already occurred, so some high-risk reperfusion strategies, such as fibrinolytic medications, carry more risk than potential benefit. As with the other ECG changes mentioned here, the absence of pathologic Q-waves does not indicate that infarction has not taken place, and may in fact be a finding early in AMI before Q-waves develop.

PATIENTS WITH NORMAL ECG OR NONDIAGNOSTIC ST/T-WAVE CHANGES

A normal ECG does not mean that the patient is not experiencing an acute coronary syndrome. These patients should undergo further evaluation before a decision is made to discharge from the acute care setting. If the patient meets criteria for new onset angina (pain persists, signs of LV dysfunction), or has cardiac markers indicative of myocardial ischemia, then he should be treated like the patient with ST depression, and receive anticoagulation, nitrates, and beta blockers. If not, serial ECGs and cardiac markers should be monitored, and clinicians may consider cardiac imaging such as echocardiography, to evaluate heart function. If there is no evidence of ischemia or injury, the patient may not receive further intervention for this event, and may be discharged, but should receive follow-up evaluation and care.

Practice Test Acute Coronary Syndromes

1. A patient on your nursing unit complains of severe substernal chest pain, 8 on a scale of 0–10. His heart rate is 110, his blood pressure is 146/88. You apply oxygen @ 2 lpm via nasal cannula, and administer 0.3 mg nitroglycerine sublingual. Three minutes later, he describes his pain as 7 on a scale of 1–10. Which pharmacologic agent should you administer next?
   A. Morphine sulfate IV.
   B. Nitroglycerine sublingual.
   C. Vasotec IV.
   D. Lopressor IV.

2. In addition to oxygen, nitroglycerine, and morphine, which agent is indicated in the initial management of the patient with ischemic chest pain?
   A. Aspirin.
   B. Demerol.

C. Norepinephrine.

D. Magnesium.

3. A 60-year-old patient complains of substernal chest pain. The 12-lead ECG show 1.5 mm ST elevation in leads II, III, and aVF. Assuming there are no contraindications to any therapy, which of the following interventions would be appropriate ?
   A. Aspirin and IV calcium channel blockers.
   B. ACE inhibitors IV and low-molecular-weight heparin
   C. Fibrinolytics and heparin.
   D. Antiarrhythmics and vasopressors.

4. ST elevation on the 12-lead ECG should make the clinician highly suspicious for:
   A. Myocardial perforation.
   B. Myocardial injury.
   C. Myocardial infarction.
   D. Myocardial ischemia.

5. The appropriate dose of oxygen for the patient with ischemic chest pain, with a heart rate of 90 bpm, BP 128/74, RR 12/min, and SaO_2 96% is:
   A. 100% via bag valve mask.
   B. Nonrebreather mask.
   C. 28% Venturi mask.
   D. 2–6 1pm via nasal cannula.

6. The patient with a non-ST segment elevation MI may receive all the following agents except:
   A. Nitroglycerine.
   B. Clopidogrel.
   C. Fibrinolytics.
   D. Glycoprotein IIb/IIIa inhibitors.

7. A 55-year-old male complains of severe chest pressure, 9 on a scale of 1–10. He reports that the pain began 20 minutes ago while he was sitting in a chair reading. He states that he has never experienced discomfort like this before and has never been told he has heart disease. He is normal weight for his height and he does not smoke. His HR is 100 bpm, BP 138/88, RR 12, SaO_2 95%. You apply oxygen 2 lpm via nasal cannula and administer aspirin 162 mg po and nitroglycerine 0.4 mg sl. Three minutes later, he rates his pain 7 on a scale of 0–10, BP 130/80, and complains of slight nausea. Which is the best next action?
   A. Administer morphine 3 mg IVP.
   B. Prepare to transfer to cardiac cath lab.
   C. Repeat nitroglycerine 0.4 mg sl.
   D. Repeat aspirin 162 mg po.

8. Minutes later, the 12-lead ECG shows ST depression and T-wave inversion in leads II, III, and aVf. Which of the following interventions is inappropriate?
   A. Begin arrangements for cardiac catheterization and possible angioplasty.
   B. Obtain consent for fibrinolytics and administer as soon as possible.
   C. Order serial 12-lead ECGs to monitor for further changes.
   D. Administer Clopidogrel 300 mg po.

9. After aspirin, 3 doses of nitroglycerine, and increase of oxygen to 6 lpm, the patient rates his pain 6 on a scale of 0–10. His heart rate is 100 bpm, BP 128/76, RR 12/min, SaO_2 97%. Which of the following agents should be administered next?
   A. Diltiazem 20 mg IVP.
   B. Furosemide 20 mg IVP.

C. Lidocaine 1.0 mg/kg IVP.
D. Morphine Sulfate 2 mg IVP.

10. Which of the following patients is most likely to have atypical or vague symptoms of an acute coronary syndrome?
    A. A 65-year-old woman with diabetes in good control.
    B. A 70-year-old man on the telemetry unit following radical prostatectomy.
    C. A 45-year-old man who smokes three packs of cigarettes per day.
    D. A 50-year-old man with a history of angina.

CHAPTER

9 ACLS Patient Management Algorithms

Putting It All Together

The final goal of any ACLS education program is to provide participants with the knowledge to manage patients displaying a variety of cardiac conditions. It must be understood that patient care is dynamic and must change as the patient's condition changes, thus the provider must have an understanding of each of ten patient management cases and have the ability to move from one condition to another.

Understanding clinical assessment, airway management, ECG interpretation, electrical therapy, and pharmacology is a must. Being able to employ these treatment modalities to manage patient cases is critical.

The following algorithm flowcharts are designed to assist in recalling the most common patient cases and complications. Utilizing a standardized approach will help with recall and decrease the likelihood of missing important steps. We have simplified the algorithms by placing each condition on one page with a linear approach for ease of recall. As the patient's condition changes, the clinician merely "changes the page" in his mind and continues to manage the specific condition.

We find the memorization easier when the patients are thought of and grouped as either perfusing (with a pulse) or arrested (without a pulse).

Tips for Managing Perfusing Patients

During an ACLS course you should generally assume your patient who is conscious and speaking will not stay that way for long so gather any information you may need early on. **Generally assessment and initial management will take place simultaneously.**

Begin with the basics of all patient care:

Assess and maintain Airway, Breathing, and Circulation.

Evaluate the patient's symptoms and related history. Begin a physical exam.

Things to do:

Administer oxygen.

Assess and monitor vital and diagnostic signs:

Respirations, pulse, B/P, pulse oximetry, monitor ECG rhythm

Establish vascular access.

Things to order:

12-lead ECG

Blood work, specifically cardiac enzymes

Chest X ray

Manage the condition based on the patient's presentation, and cardiovascular findings, as well as the diagnostic tools, i.e., treat the patient, not merely the monitors.

Tips for Managing Cardiac Arrested Patients

Determine the patient is unresponsive and call for "code team" support.

Employ the primary and secondary A B C D approach.

PRIMARY A B C D

A Airway—open it by placing the patient in the sniffing position.

B Breathing—assess breathing for up to 10 sec. If breathing is absent provide two breaths over 1 sec each. Use oxygen via bag valve mask, then continue one breath approximately every 6 sec (about 10/min).

C Circulation—evaluate for signs of a pulse. If pulse is absent begin and maintain compressions at 100/min. Initially use a 30-compression/2-breath ratio until an advanced airway is placed.

E Defibrillator—bring and attach a monitor/defibrillator to the patient. Shock when appropriate.

Continual high-quality chest compressions are critical.

SECONDARY A B C D

A Advanced airway procedures. Reserved for those skilled at this procedure—tracheal, esophageal or laryngeal tube. Otherwise continue with a bag valve mask.

B Breathing assessed, assured, and secured. Be sure whichever tube is placed causes chest rise. Apply supplemental O_2, then secure the device. Once the tube is placed, CPR can be performed with continual compressions at 100/min with one breath imposed every 6 sec (about 10/min)

C Circulatory interventions. Establish or confirm vascular access and begin cardiac pharmacology. *Hint:* In cardiac arrest the first medication is always a vasopressor such as epinephrine or vasopressin. Then continue epinephrine each 3–5 min.

D Differential diagnosis. Search for reversible causes if management according to the standard algorithm is not yielding a successful resuscitation.

Potential reversible causes of cardiac arrest:

Hypoxia	Toxins (overdose)
Hypovolemia	Thromboemboli (pulmonary / coronary)
Hyper/hypokalemia	Trauma
Hypothermia	Tension pneumothorax
Hydrogen ion (acidosis)	Tamponade (cardiac)
Hypoglycemia	Too fast or too slow

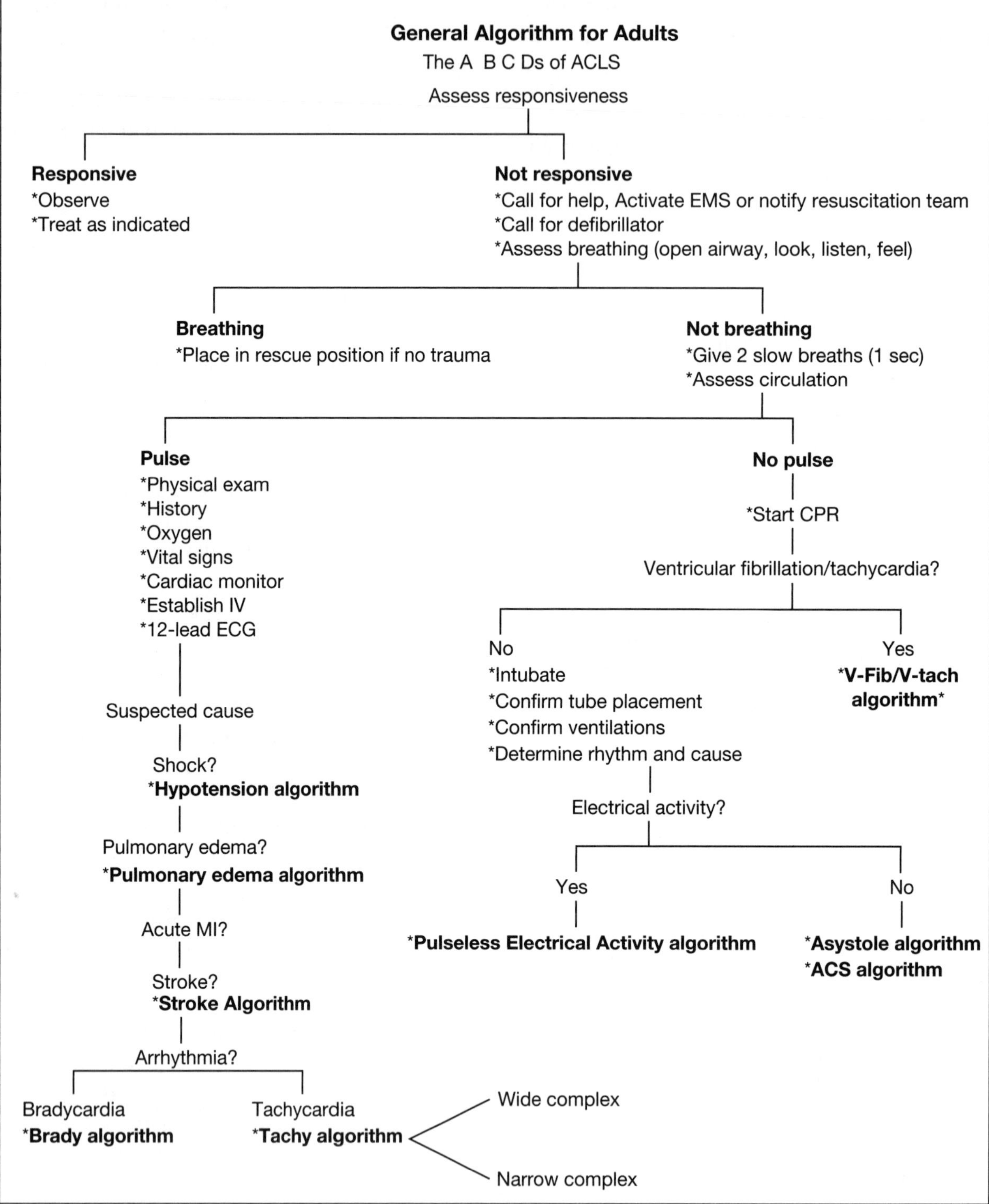
General Algorithm for Adults
The A B C Ds of ACLS
Assess responsiveness
Responsive
*Observe
*Treat as indicated
Not responsive
*Call for help, Activate EMS or notify resuscitation team
*Call for defibrillator
*Assess breathing (open airway, look, listen, feel)
Breathing
*Place in rescue position if no trauma
Not breathing
*Give 2 slow breaths (1 sec)
*Assess circulation
Pulse
*Physical exam
*History
*Oxygen
*Vital signs
*Cardiac monitor
*Establish IV
*12-lead ECG
Suspected cause
Shock?
*Hypotension algorithm
Pulmonary edema?
*Pulmonary edema algorithm
Acute MI?
Stroke?
*Stroke Algorithm
Arrhythmia?
Bradycardia
*Brady algorithm
Tachycardia
*Tachy algorithm
Wide complex
Narrow complex
No pulse
*Start CPR
Ventricular fibrillation/tachycardia?
No
*Intubate
*Confirm tube placement
*Confirm ventilations
*Determine rhythm and cause
Yes
V-Fib/V-tach algorithm
Electrical activity?
Yes
*Pulseless Electrical Activity algorithm
No
*Asystole algorithm
*ACS algorithm

Tips for Postresuscitative Care

Patients who respond positively and are resuscitated should be managed with the following in mind. The object is to improve and maintain cardiac output with an emphasis on supplying a blood pressure adequate to perfuse vital organs, generally a systolic blood pressure of 90 mm Hg.

To that end, manage postresuscitative cases in the following order:

1. Continue appropriate oxygenation and ventilation.
2. Stabilize the rate. This generally means maintaining the heart rate above 60 bpm.
3. Stabilize the rhythm. If the patient was in ventricular fibrillation or ventricular tachycardia, some will choose to administer an infusion of the antiarrhythmic that was used during the arrest. This often is physician preference.
4. Stabilize the blood pressure. Utilize fluid boluses initially. If fluids fail to provide an adequate blood pressure (90 mm Hg systolic), a vasoactive infusion such as Dopamine or Levophed should be administered.

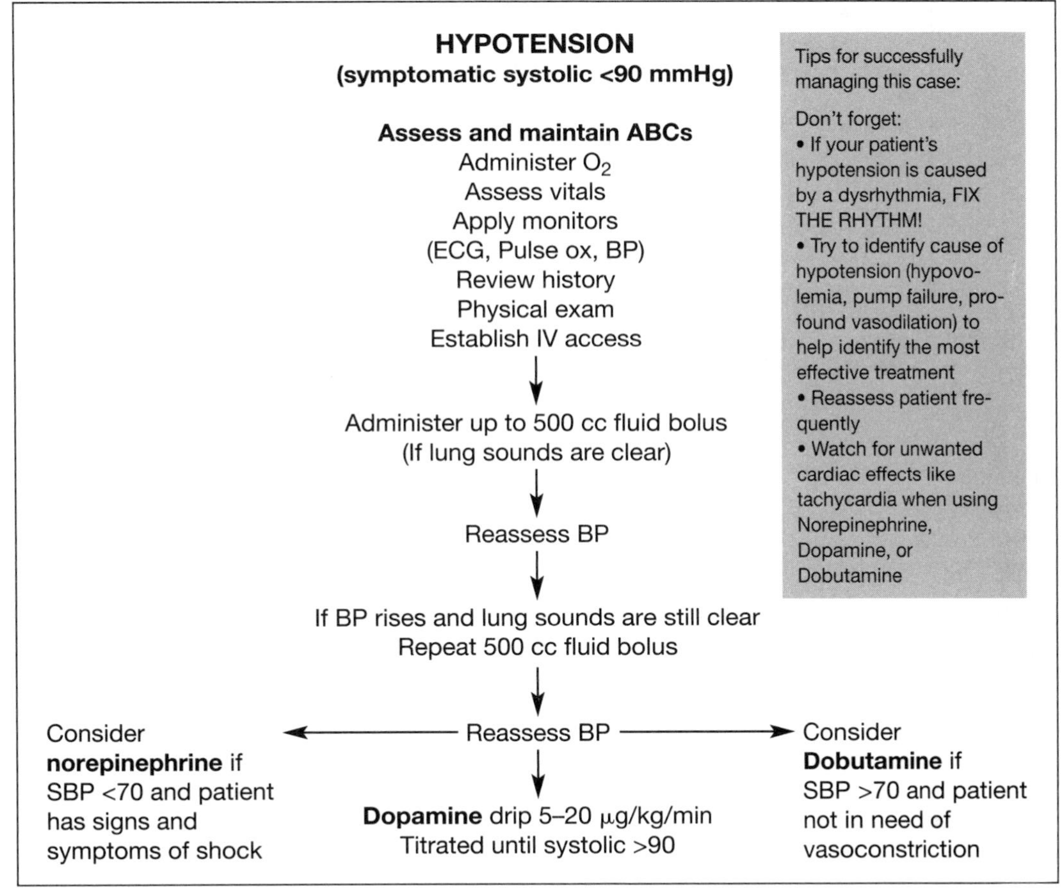

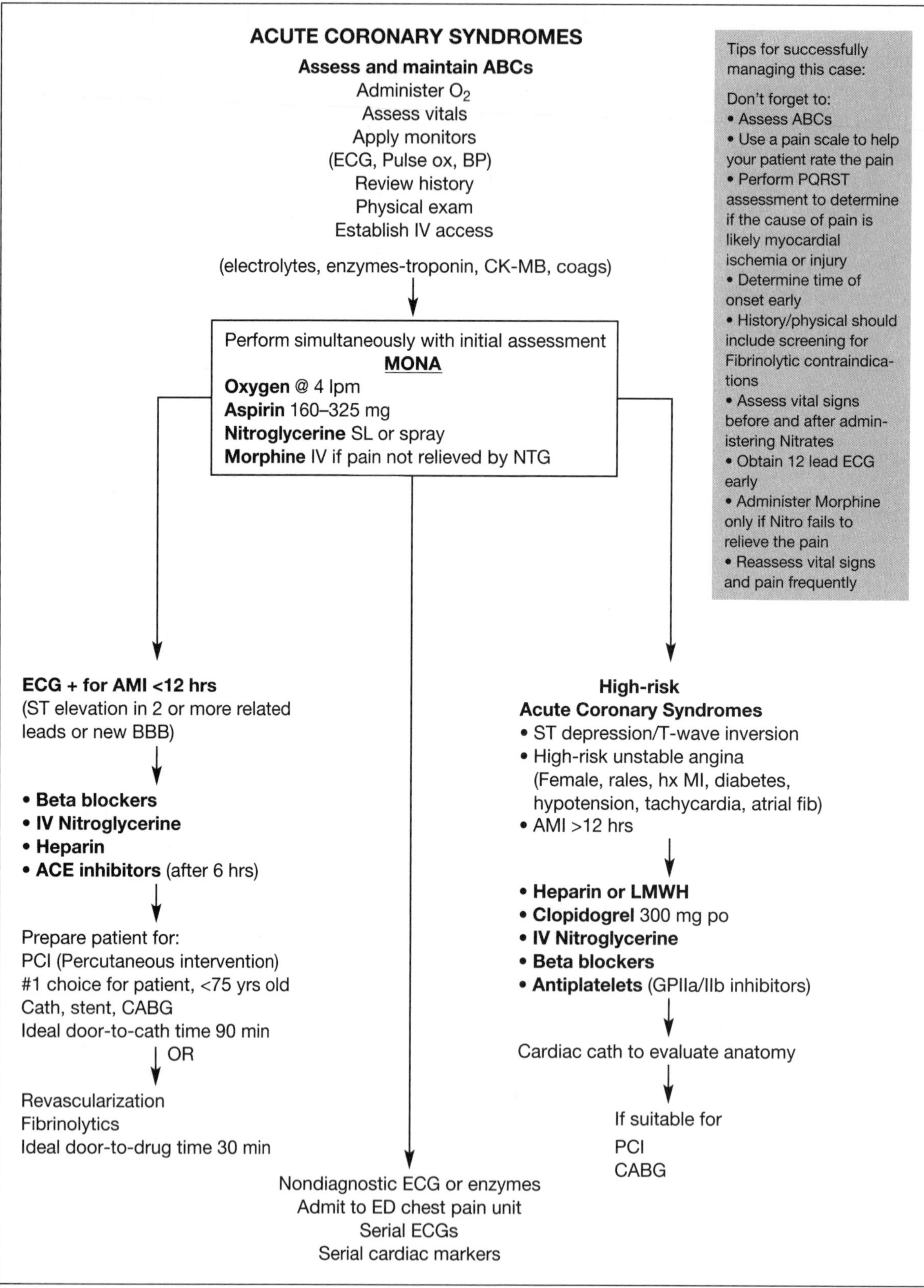
ACUTE CORONARY SYNDROMES
Assess and maintain ABCs
Administer O_2
Assess vitals
Apply monitors
(ECG, Pulse ox, BP)
Review history
Physical exam
Establish IV access
(electrolytes, enzymes-troponin, CK-MB, coags)
Perform simultaneously with initial assessment
MONA
Oxygen @ 4 lpm
Aspirin 160–325 mg
Nitroglycerine SL or spray
Morphine IV if pain not relieved by NTG
Tips for successfully managing this case:
Don't forget to:
• Assess ABCs
• Use a pain scale to help your patient rate the pain
• Perform PQRST assessment to determine if the cause of pain is likely myocardial ischemia or injury
• Determine time of onset early
• History/physical should include screening for Fibrinolytic contraindications
• Assess vital signs before and after administering Nitrates
• Obtain 12 lead ECG early
• Administer Morphine only if Nitro fails to relieve the pain
• Reassess vital signs and pain frequently
ECG + for AMI <12 hrs
(ST elevation in 2 or more related leads or new BBB)
• Beta blockers
• IV Nitroglycerine
• Heparin
• ACE inhibitors (after 6 hrs)
Prepare patient for:
PCI (Percutaneous intervention)
#1 choice for patient, <75 yrs old
Cath, stent, CABG
Ideal door-to-cath time 90 min
OR
Revascularization
Fibrinolytics
Ideal door-to-drug time 30 min
High-risk
Acute Coronary Syndromes
• ST depression/T-wave inversion
• High-risk unstable angina
(Female, rales, hx MI, diabetes, hypotension, tachycardia, atrial fib)
• AMI >12 hrs
• Heparin or LMWH
• Clopidogrel 300 mg po
• IV Nitroglycerine
• Beta blockers
• Antiplatelets (GPIIa/IIb inhibitors)
Cardiac cath to evaluate anatomy
If suitable for
PCI
CABG
Nondiagnostic ECG or enzymes
Admit to ED chest pain unit
Serial ECGs
Serial cardiac markers

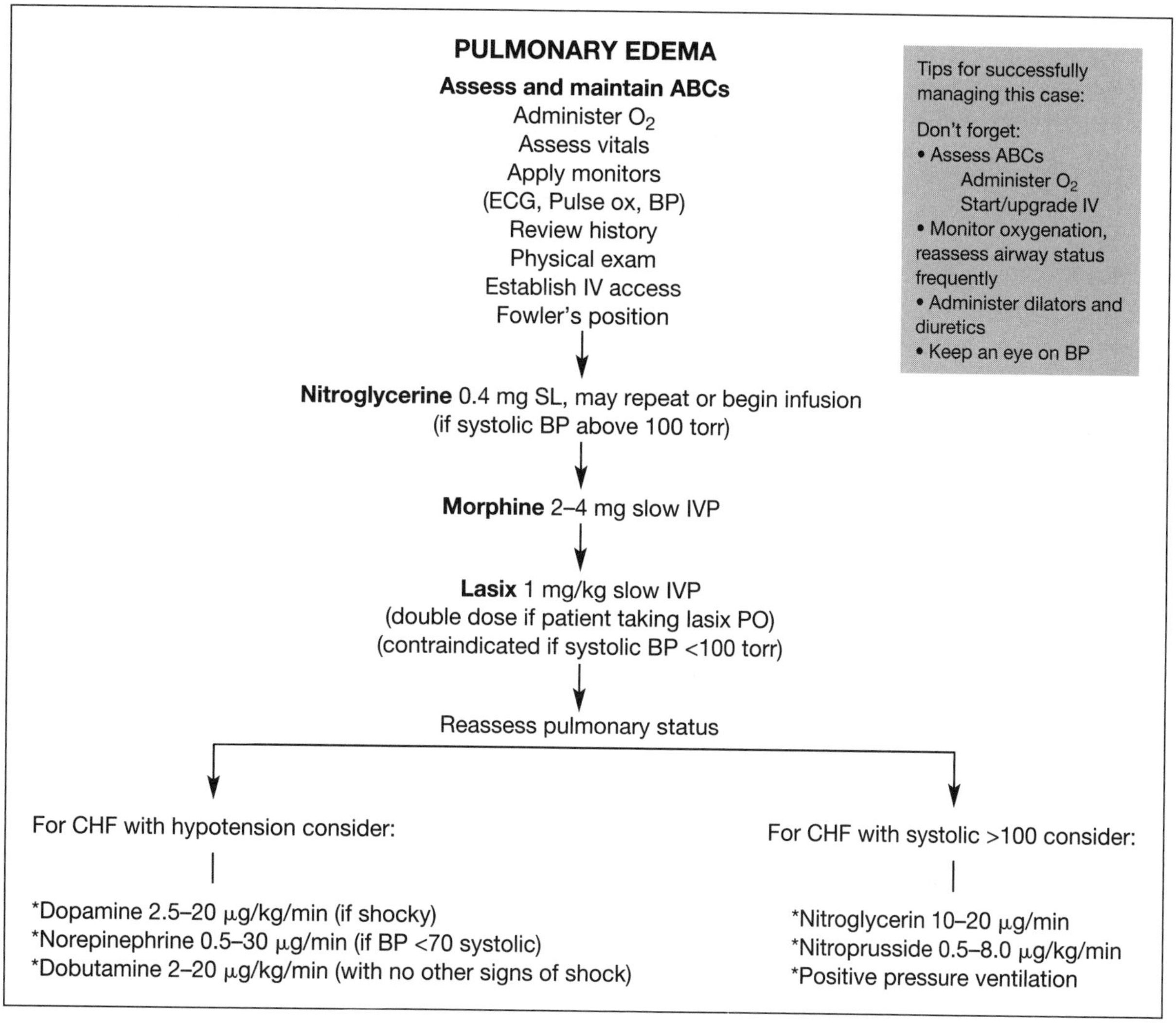

PULMONARY EDEMA

Assess and maintain ABCs
Administer O_2
Assess vitals
Apply monitors
(ECG, Pulse ox, BP)
Review history
Physical exam
Establish IV access
Fowler's position

↓

Nitroglycerine 0.4 mg SL, may repeat or begin infusion
(if systolic BP above 100 torr)

↓

Morphine 2–4 mg slow IVP

↓

Lasix 1 mg/kg slow IVP
(double dose if patient taking lasix PO)
(contraindicated if systolic BP <100 torr)

↓

Reassess pulmonary status

For CHF with hypotension consider:

*Dopamine 2.5–20 μg/kg/min (if shocky)
*Norepinephrine 0.5–30 μg/min (if BP <70 systolic)
*Dobutamine 2–20 μg/kg/min (with no other signs of shock)

For CHF with systolic >100 consider:

*Nitroglycerin 10–20 μg/min
*Nitroprusside 0.5–8.0 μg/kg/min
*Positive pressure ventilation

Tips for successfully managing this case:

Don't forget:
- Assess ABCs
  Administer O_2
  Start/upgrade IV
- Monitor oxygenation, reassess airway status frequently
- Administer dilators and diuretics
- Keep an eye on BP

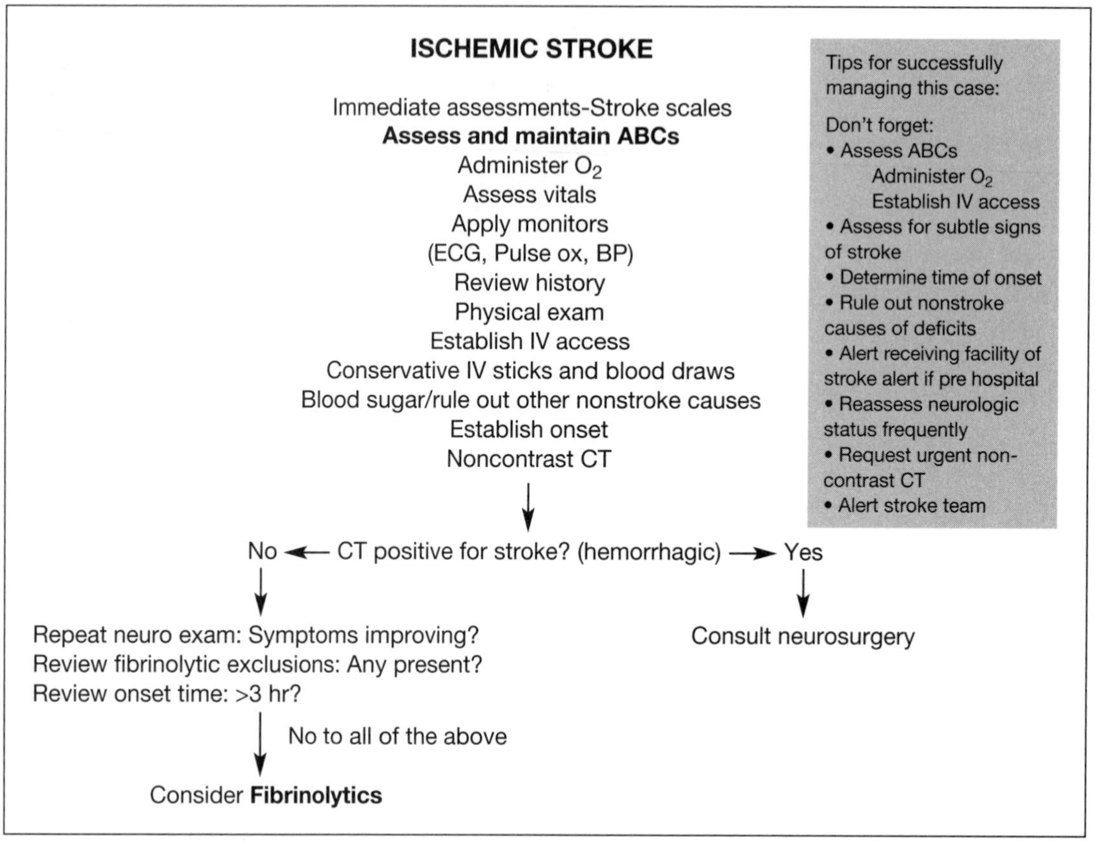

ISCHEMIC STROKE

Immediate assessments-Stroke scales
Assess and maintain ABCs
Administer O_2
Assess vitals
Apply monitors
(ECG, Pulse ox, BP)
Review history
Physical exam
Establish IV access
Conservative IV sticks and blood draws
Blood sugar/rule out other nonstroke causes
Establish onset
Noncontrast CT

↓

No ← CT positive for stroke? (hemorrhagic) → Yes

Yes ↓ Consult neurosurgery

No ↓
Repeat neuro exam: Symptoms improving?
Review fibrinolytic exclusions: Any present?
Review onset time: >3 hr?

↓ No to all of the above

Consider **Fibrinolytics**

Tips for successfully managing this case:

Don't forget:
- Assess ABCs
  Administer O_2
  Establish IV access
- Assess for subtle signs of stroke
- Determine time of onset
- Rule out nonstroke causes of deficits
- Alert receiving facility of stroke alert if pre hospital
- Reassess neurologic status frequently
- Request urgent non-contrast CT
- Alert stroke team

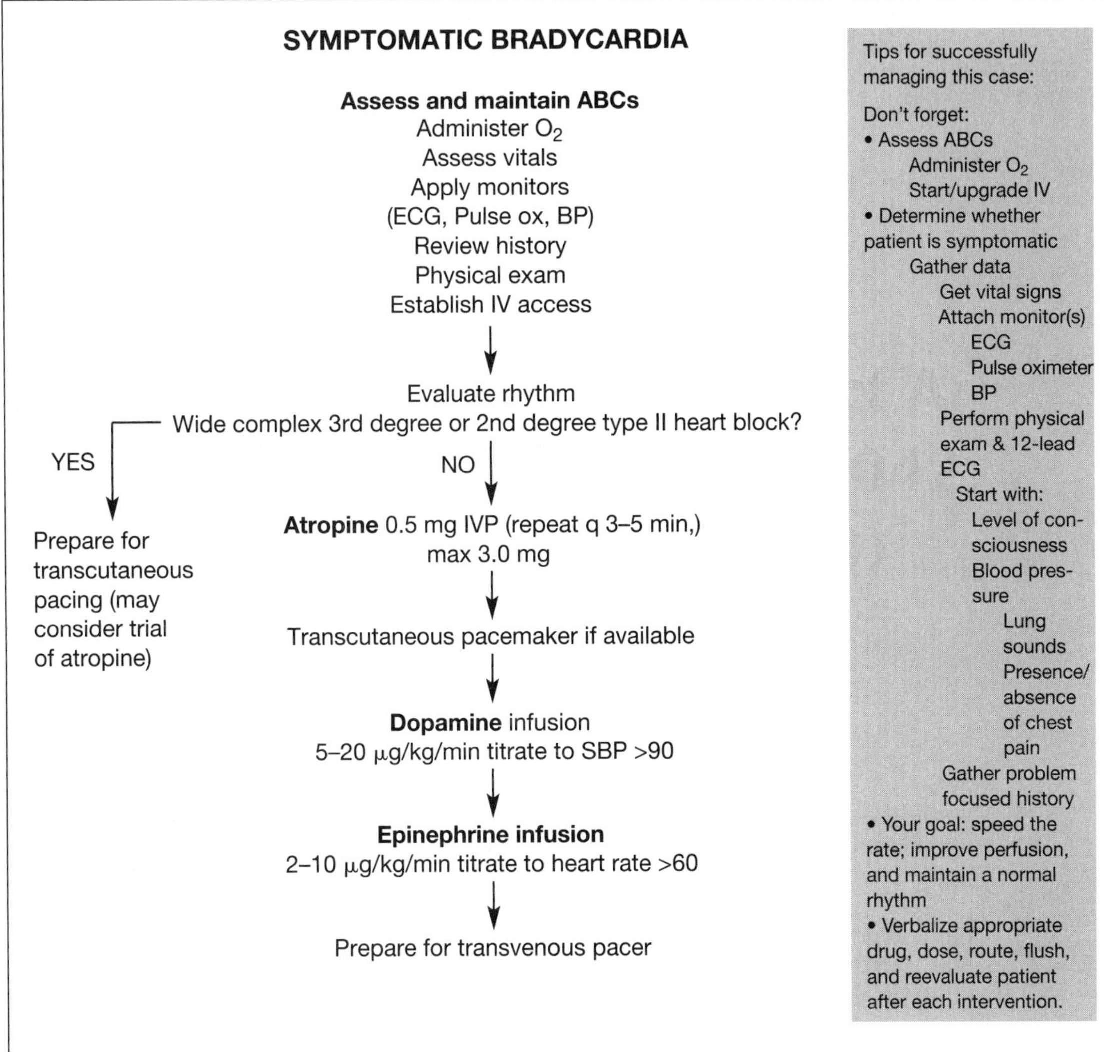

Quick Tip

When treating bradycardia, remember, "**A**fter **t**en **d**on't **e**at" (Atropine, transcutaneous pacing, dopamine, epinephrine)

SUPRAVENTRICULAR TACHYCARDIA, STABLE

(Maintaining adequate mentation, blood pressure, respiratory status, and absence of chest pain)

Narrow complex, rate over 150, regular with no P-waves or signs of A-fib or flutter

Assess and maintain ABCs

Administer O_2
Assess vitals
Apply monitors
(ECG, Pulse ox, BP)
Review history
Physical exam
Establish IV access → Atrial fib/flutter? See AF algorithm

Consider ordering:
(12-lead ECG, cardiac enzymes, CXR)
(Expert cardiology consult).

↓

Vagal Maneuvers

↓

Adenosine 6 mg IVP rapidly followed by flush
Adenosine 12 mg IVP rapidly followed by flush
May repeat Adenosine 12 mg ×1

If rhythm fails to convert
Choose one:

Calcium Channel Blocker
Diltiazem 15–20 mg may repeat 20–25 mg in 15 min
Verapamil 2.5–5.0 mg may repeat 5–10 mg in 15–30 min
OR
Beta blocker
Atenolol 5 mg over 5 min may repeat in 10 min
Metoprolol 5 mg over 5 min may repeat Q5 ×2

↓

If rhythm still fails to convert

May choose sedation and elective cardioversion or other medications based on a more definitive rhythm diagnosis.

Tips for successfully managing this case:

Don't forget:
- Assess ABCs
  - Administer O_2
  - Start/upgrade IV
- Determine whether patient is stable or unstable
  - Gather data
    - Get vital signs
    - Attach monitor(s)
      - ECG
      - Pulse oximeter
      - BP
  - Perform physical exam & 12 lead ECG
    - Start with:
      - Level of consciousness
      - Blood pressure
        - Lung sounds
        - Presence/absence of chest pain
  - Gather problem focused history
- Your goal: slow the rate; improve perfusion and maintain a normal rhythm
- Verbalize appropriate drug, dose, route, flush, and reevaluate patient after each intervention.

SUPRAVENTRICULAR TACHYCARDIA
ATRIAL FIBRILLATION/FLUTTER, STABLE WITH RAPID VENTRICULAR RESPONSE
Sustained rate over 150
(Maintaining adequate mentation, blood pressure, respiratory status, and absence of chest pain)

Assess and maintain ABCs
Administer O_2
Assess vitals
Apply monitors
(ECG, Pulse ox, BP)
Review history
Physical exam
Establish IV access

Consider ordering:
(12-lead ECG, cardiac enzymes, CXR)
(Expert cardiology consult).

↓

Control rate with:
Choose one:

Calcium Channel Blocker
Diltiazem 15–20 mg may repeat 20–25 mg in 15 min
Verapamil 2.5–5.0 mg may repeat 5–10 mg in 15–30 min
OR
Beta blocker
Atenolol 5 mg over 5 min may repeat in 10 min
Metoprolol 5 mg over 5 min may repeat Q5 × 2
OR
Magnesium 1–2 grams over 5–60 min

Convert rhythm after expert cardiology consult?
Duration of fib flutter?

<48 hr

Convert rhythm by the same means as the patient who has had emboli ruled out up to 4 weeks

For conversion:

>48 hr

Delay rhythm <u>conversion</u> unless unstable:

- R/O emboli or anticoagulation
- May use any one of the following

1. Elective cardioversion. May start 50 J for A-flutter.
2. Amiodarone 150 mg over 10 min then infusion.
3. Ibulitide 1.0 mg over 10 min may repeat in 10 min.
4. Digitalis 10–15 μg/kg (0.5–1.0 mg)

Tips for successfully managing this case:

Don't forget:
- Assess ABCs
  - Administer O_2
  - Start/upgrade IV
- Determine whether patient is symptomatic due to the *heart rate:*
  - Gather data ESPECIALLY ONSET TIME
    - Get vital signs
    - Attach monitor(s)
      - ECG
      - Pulse oximeter
      - BP
  - Perform physical exam & 12-lead ECG
    - Start with:
      - Level of consciousness
      - Blood pressure
        - Lung sounds
        - Presence/absence of chest pain
  - Gather problem focused history
  - Rule out non cardiac causes.
- Your goal: slow the rate; improve perfusion
- Verbalize appropriate drug, dose, route, flush, and reevaluate patient after each intervention.

UNSTABLE TACHYCARDIA OF ANY TYPE
(WIDE OR NARROW COMPLEX)
Rate over 150 with decreased LOC, hypotension, pulmonary edema, or chest pain

Assess and support ABCDs
Administer O_2
Assess vitals
Apply monitors

↓

(ECG, Pulse ox, BP)
Brief history
IV/IO access
(Do not delay cardioversion for IV)

↓

Immediate management
Sedation
(If conscious and B/P allows)

↓

Synchronized cardioversion
100 j, 200 j, 300 j, 360 j
(Or biphasic equivalent usually 120–200 j)

If unsuccessful:
medication sequence for stable

Tips for successfully managing this case:

Don't forget:
- Assess ABCs
  - Administer O_2
  - Start/upgrade IV
- Determine whether patient is stable or unstable
  - Gather data
    - Get vital signs
    - Attach monitor(s)
      - ECG
      - Pulse oximeter
      - BP
  - Start with:
    - Level of consciousness
    - Blood pressure
      - Lung sounds
      - Presence/absence of chest pain
  - Gather problem focused history
- Your goal: slow the rate; improve perfusion and maintain a normal rhythm
- Verbalize appropriate drug, dose, route, flush, and reevaluate patient after each intervention.

Quick Tip

Tachycardia and awake (or otherwise stable), then we are to medicate.

Tachycardia with a nap (or otherwise unstable), then the treatment's Zap Zap Zap!

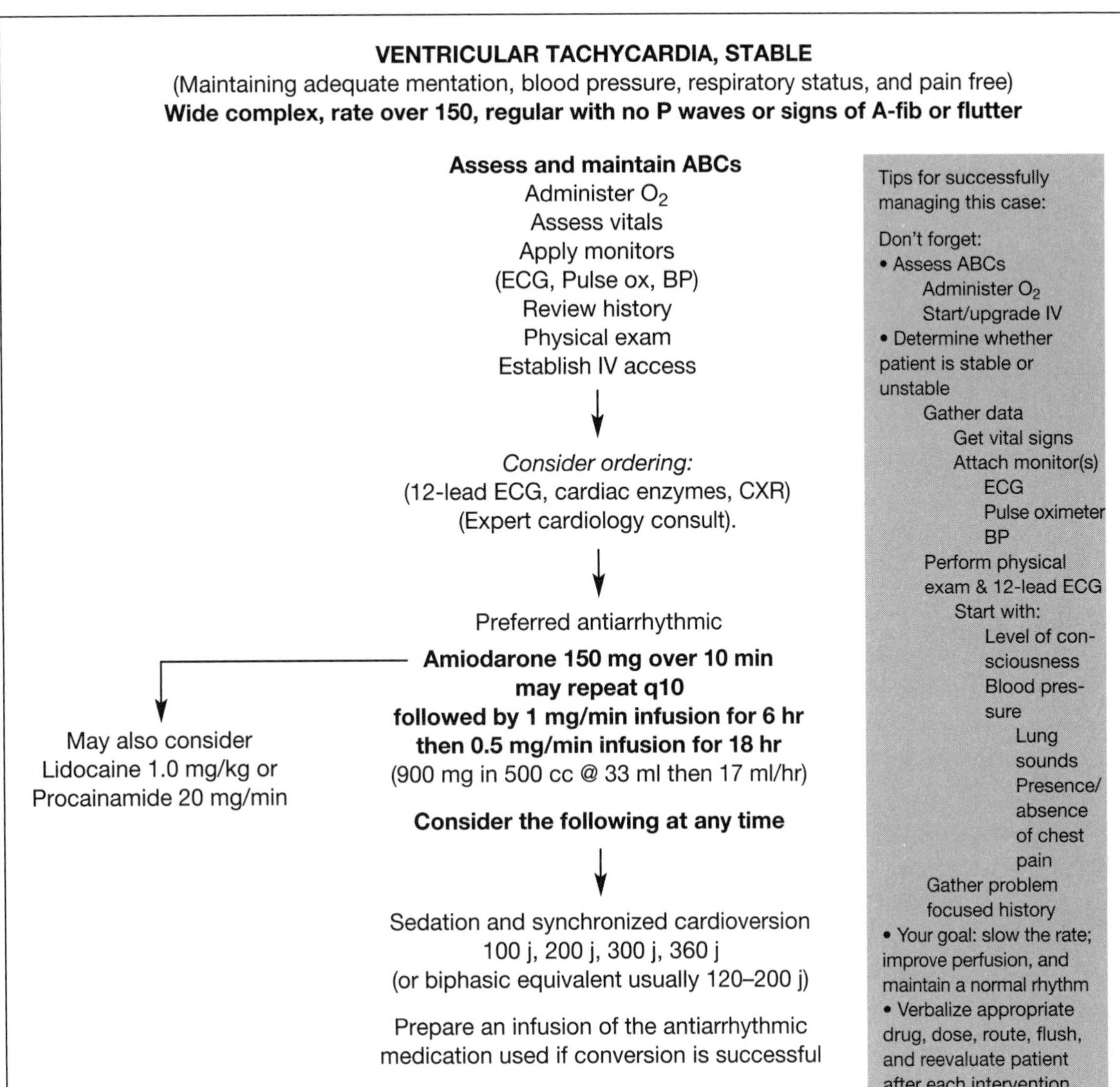

Quick Tip

Find the cause! Patients don't have ventricular tach because they are low on lidocaine (or any other antiarrhythmic). Medications are a temporary Band-Aid for ventricular irritability, but it is likely to recur if the cause is not diagnosed and treated.

VENTRICULAR FIBRILLATION
or
PULSELESS VENTRICULAR TACHYCARDIA

ABCDs

Perform CPR until defibrillator available
If unwitnessed (EMS) perform CPR 2 min then defibrillate
If witnessed defibrillate when available

Defibrillate 200 j or device-specific dose
Continue CPR 2 min

Reassess. If still VF, defibrillate 200–360 j or device specific dose. Resume CPR for 2 min

Secure airway
Establish IV or IO with NS or LR

Vasopressor of choice
given during CPR
Epinephrine 1.0 mg
OR
Vasopressin 40 u ×1
instead of 1st or 2nd epi dose
Then revert to epinephrine

Defibrillate 200 j–360 j or device-specific dose
Continue CPR 2 min

Antiarrhythmic of choice
given during CPR
Amiodarone 300 mg
OR
Lidocaine 1.0–1.5 mg/kg (If Amiodarone not available)

Defibrillate 200 j–360 j or device-specific dose

Repeat sequence of CPR 2 min—One medication—Defibrillate

Repeat epinephrine q 3 min

Repeat Amiodarone 150 mg ×1 or

Lidocaine 0.5–0.75 mg/kg up to 3 mg/kg max (If Lidocaine was used)

Evaluate for and treat reversible causes anytime during the sequence:

Hypoxia	**T**oxins (overdose)
Hypovolemia	**T**hromboemboli (pulmonary/coronary)
Hyper/hypokalemia	**T**rauma
Hypothermia	**T**ension pneumothorax
Hydrogen ion (acidosis)	**T**amponade (cardiac)
Hypoglycemia	**T**oo fast or too slow

Tips for successfully managing this case:

Don't forget:
- Assess ABCs
  - Continue CPR throughout and for 2 min between shocks
  - No rush to intubate
  - Start/upgrade IV or IO Gather focused history

Primary goal: continue effective CPR followed by rotating medications and defibrillation attempts.
- Verbalize appropriate drug, dose, route, flush, and reevaluate patient each 2 minutes.

Once a rhythm is restored, maintain ventilations as appropriate then stabilize in order:
1. Rate
2. Rhythm
3. Blood pressure

Quick Tip

The sequence rotates CPR—Drug—Shock with an emphasis on continual, good CPR.

PULSELESS ELECTRICAL ACTIVITY

ABCDs
Perform CPR
Secure airway
Establish IV or IO with NS or LR

↓

Vasopressor of choice
given during CPR
Epinephrine 1.0 mg
OR
Vasopressin 40 u ×1
instead of 1st or 2nd epi dose
Then revert to epinephrine q 3–5 min

↓

If ventricular rate <60/min
Atropine 1 mg
q 3–5 min to max of 3 mg

↓

Continue CPR and medication rotation while searching for the reversible causes:

Evaluate for and treat reversible causes anytime during the sequence:

Hypoxia	**T**oxins (overdose)
Hypovolemia	**T**hromboemboli (pulmonary/coronary)
Hyper/hypokalemia	**T**rauma
Hypothermia	**T**ension pneumothorax
Hydrogen ion (acidosis)	**T**amponade (cardiac)
Hypoglycemia	**T**oo fast or too slow

Tips for successfully managing this case:

Don't forget:
- Assess ABCs
  - Continue CPR throughout, 2 min between assessments.
  - No rush to intubate
  - Start/upgrade IV or IO
  - Gather focused history

Primary goal: continue effective CPR followed by medications and determining the cause (H's & T's).
- Verbalize appropriate drug, dose, route, flush, and reevaluate patient after each intervention.

Once a rhythm is restored, maintain ventilations as appropriate then stabilize in order:
1. Rate
2. Rhythm
3. Blood pressure

Quick Tip

To treat PEA, **P**ush **E**pi **A**nd… consider the causes

ASYSTOLE

ABCDs
Perform CPR
Check equipment, cables, electrodes, check gain
Confirm asystole in more than 1 lead

↓

Secure airway
Establish IV or IO with NS or LR

↓

Vasopressor of choice
given during CPR
Epinephrine 1.0 mg
OR
Vasopressin 40 u × 1
instead of 1st or 2nd epi dose
Then revert to epinephrine q 3–5 min

↓

Atropine 1.0 mg
given during CPR
Repeat q 3–5 min
to max total dose 3 mg

↓

Evaluate for and treat reversible causes anytime during the sequence:

Hypoxia	**T**oxins (overdose)
Hypovolemia	**T**hromboemboli (pulmonary/coronary)
Hyper/hypokalemia	**T**rauma
Hypothermia	**T**ension pneumothorax
Hydrogen ion (acidosis)	**T**amponade (cardiac)
Hypoglycemia	**T**oo fast or too slow

↓

If patient remains in asystole or other agonal rhythms after successful airway control and initial medications and no reversible causes are identified, consider termination of resuscitative efforts.

Tips for successfully managing this case:

Don't forget:
- Assess ABCs
  Continue CPR throughout, 2 min between assessments.
  No rush to intubate
  Start/upgrade IV or IO
  Gather focused history

Primary goal: continue effective CPR followed by medications and determining the cause (H's & T's).
- Verbalize appropriate drug, dose, route, flush, and reevaluate patient after each intervention.

Once a rhythm is restored, maintain ventilations as appropriate, then stabilize in order:
1. Rate
2. Rhythm
3. Blood pressure

Quick Tip

To work on asystole think DEAD—
Do CPR, **E**pi, **A**tropine, ***D***o it again.

INCLUSION/EXCLUSION CRITERIA FOR FIBRINOLYTIC THERAPY

CARDIAC

Inclusion Criteria

[ ] Chest pain and/or symptoms of acute MI
[ ] QRS duration <120 ms (0.12 sec)
[ ] ST segment elevation > 0.1 mv (1 mm)
 [ ] In 2 or more leads
 [ ] II, III, aVF
 [ ] V1, V2, V3, V4, V5, V6
 [ ] I, aVL

Exclusion Criteria

[ ] Active internal bleeding
[ ] History of CVA/TIA

Recent (<2 months)

[ ] Intracranial/intraspinal surgery/trauma
[ ] Brain tumor, aneurysm
[ ] Arteriovenous malformation
[ ] Bleeding disorder/anticoagulant

Recent (<2 weeks)

[ ] Major surgery
[ ] Trauma
[ ] Organ biopsy
[ ] GI or GU bleeding
[ ] Severe uncontrolled HTN (200/120)
[ ] Pregnancy/Menses
[ ] Diabetic eye problems and/or other hemorrhagic opthalmic condition
[ ] Disoriented, uncooperative
[ ] Prolonged/traumatic CPR
[ ] Aortic dissection
[ ] Allergy to streptokinase

STROKE

Inclusion Criteria (Abnormal Findings)

Facial droop (*patient shows teeth or smiles*)
[ ] Normal (*both sides of face move equally well*)
[ ] Abnormal (*one side of face doesn't move as well as the other side*)

Arm Drift:
[ ] Normal (*both arms move the same OR both arms don't move at all*)
[ ] Abnormal (*one arm either doesn't move OR one arm drifts down compared to the other*)

Speech: (*The patient says, "The sky is blue in Cincinnati"*)
[ ] Normal (*patient says correct words with no slurring of words*)
[ ] Abnormal (*patient slurs words, says the wrong words, or is unable to speak*)

This scale should not be done on:
- Multiple trauma victims (e.g., car accidents, assaults, gunshot wounds)
- Isolated minor injuries (e.g., twisted ankles, sore throats, toothaches, simple lacerations)
- Critically ill patients (e.g., BP >80, intubated patients)

Exclusion Criteria

- Stroke>3.0 hours old
- Seizure prior to the onset of stroke symptoms
- A prior stroke or serious head injury within 3 months
- Major surgery within 14 days
- Known history of intracranial hemorrhage
- GI or GU hemorrhage within 21 days

Note: If prehospital personnel are unsure of time of onset or whether patient meets exclusion criteria, they should initiate "STROKE ALERT" and allow Emergency Department to make decision.

CHAPTER

10 Tips for the Expert

This section if generally not considered part of the standard ACLS Course. The information contained herein is designed for those who seek a deeper knowledge of unique cases and more in-depth issues relating to cardiac care. The goal is to provide some "outside the box" thinking for those who may be charged with the task of making decisions during the course of patient management.

Advanced Issues in Basic Life Support

ALTERNATIVE CPR TECHNIQUES

Following are alternative CPR techniques to use:

High-frequency Chest Compressions

The use of high-frequency chest compressions is a technique that may be considered by clinicians, although it has not been studied thoroughly enough to receive a recommendation from international experts. Some evidence suggests that compression rates greater than 100/min produced better blood flow than conventional CPR. It is important to remember that whichever compression rate is chosen, adequate compression depth, enough to produce blood movement, is essential. Additionally, current CPR guidelines recommend changing compressors every 2 minutes to avoid decreasing effectiveness of compressions due to fatigue.

Interposed Abdominal Compressions

In settings such as hospitals, where many rescuers are available, the team may elect to perform interposed abdominal compressions. The procedure requires one or more rescuers at the head for airway management, one compressor at the classic site for chest compressions, and one rescuer to provide abdominal compressions during the "release" or relaxation phase of the chest compressions. The abdominal compressions appear to enhance venous return, better filling the heart during CPR. This combination of chest and abdominal compressions can also be achieved with a handheld device that alternates chest compressions and abdominal compressions.

Active Compression-Decompression CPR

Compression-decompression CPR uses a plunger-like device to compress the chest, then pull it back out before the next compression. The decompression phase is thought to increase venous return to the heart. One study showed an increased incidence of sternal fractures when this device was used, and other studies showed that adequate training and practice played a large role in providers being able to use the device effectively. Research supports the use of this technique in hospital settings where personnel are trained to use it.

Vest CPR

A chest encircling band attached to a backboard that rhythmically constricts provides better outcomes from cardiac arrest in some studies. Concerns such as compressor fatigue are lessened when the compressions are provided mechanically. Like other CPR devices, the successful use of the device depends on qualified users, so wherever these devices are available, frequent training and practice should occur.

Impedance Threshold Devices

A one-way valve type unit can be attached to the ventilation device (i.e., tracheal tube) to prevent air return into the lungs during the relaxation phase of chest compressions. This seems to reduce the effects of a maintained positive pressure within the thoracic cavity. Positive intrathoracic pressure has been associated with a decrease in the coronary blood flow. Hence, this device may make CPR compressions more effective, yielding better circulation.

Advanced Issues in Airway Management

While there is no science to show that intubation affects survivability from cardiac arrest, and the ACLS literature states that bag valve mask, esophageal, and laryngeal airways are all acceptable and effective depending on the skill level of the provider, clinically endotracheal intubation is the most commonly performed advanced airway skill.

To that end, this section discusses some techniques for placing an endotracheal tube in the difficult patient.

POSITIONING

1. Elevate the occiput using a towel prior to placing the patient in the sniffing position. This actually aligns the axes of intubation more effectively in many patients (Figure 10-1).

FIGURE 10-1 Occiput elevated prior to intubation (Photo: Shaun Fix, Emergency Medical Consultants.)

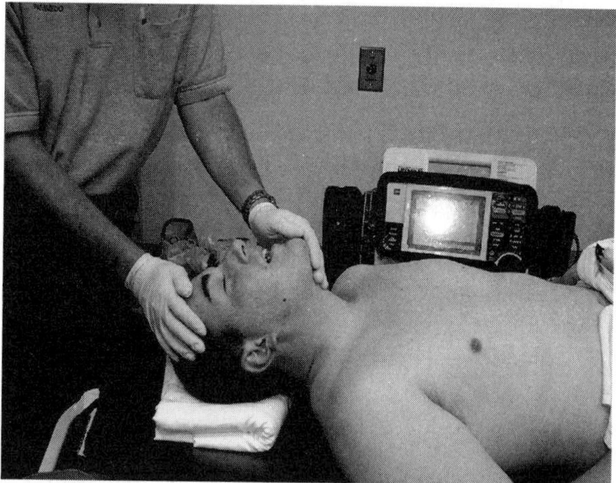

FIGURE 10-2 Intubation from the semi-fowler's position. (Photo: Shaun Fix, Emergency Medical Consultants, Inc.)

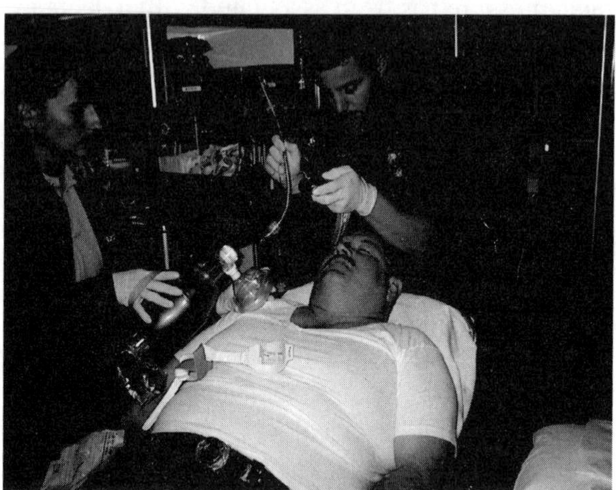

FIGURE 10-3 Bougie-intubating stylette in place

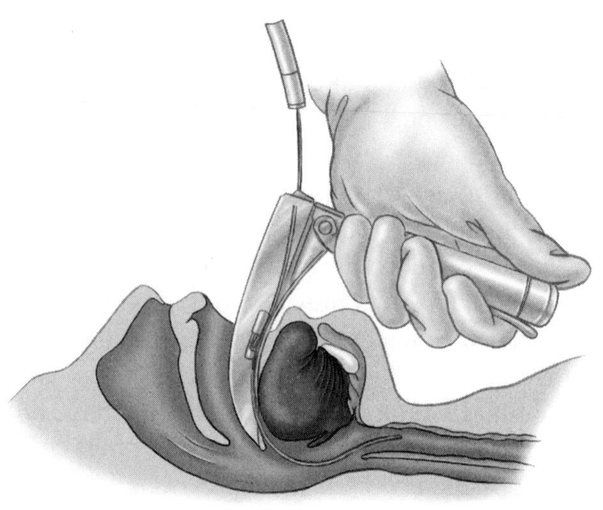

2. Place the patient in the semi-fowler's position and lower. This moves the anatomy downward thus out of the field of view and places the intubator above the patient allowing you to "look down" the patient's throat to perform the intubation (Figure 10-2).

Several commercial devices provide rapid access to controlled ventilation by way of a cuffed end isolating the larynx. Following effective ventilation these devices allow for an endotracheal tube to be passed through the device and into the trachea. Two such devices are pictured in Figure 10-4b.

EQUIPMENT

1. Bougie-intubating stylette (Figure 10-3). This plastic stylette is utilized for cases when visualization of the glottic opening is not possible. The device is used to "feel" your way into the trachea, by visualizing as much of the epiglottis as possible using the standard laryngoscope. Following this visualization the bougie is gently slid up and under the epiglottis and into the trachea. The tracheal rings will be felt as "clicking" as the bougie stylette enters the trachea. This then acts as a guide wire over which the tracheal tube is passed blindly into the trachea.
2. Intubation via a laryngeal ventilation device, which allows for intubation following ventilations (Figure 10-4a).

FIGURE 10-4a Intubating laryngeal mask airway

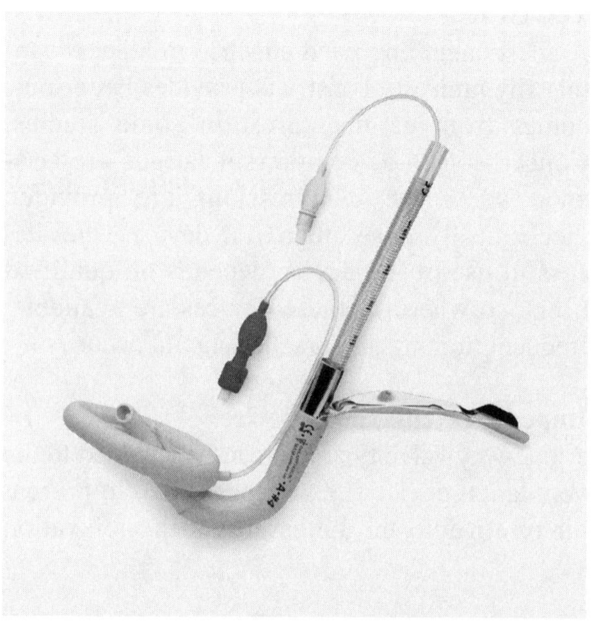

FIGURE 10-4b Perilaryngeal airway

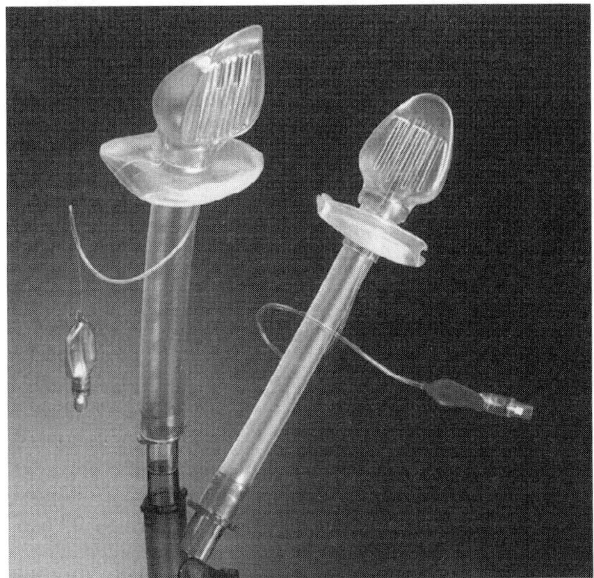

Advanced Topics in Rhythm Recognition

TORSADES DE POINTES

Torsades de pointes, or polymorphic ventricular tachycardia, is a potentially lethal arrhythmia that you should learn to recognize once you have a grasp of basic rhythm recognition. Torsades has a trademark appearance and often occurs as an end result of the lengthening of the QT interval. This abnormally long QT interval can be caused by electrolyte imbalance (often magnesium), medications, ischemia or infarction, or acute changes in intracranial pressure (Figure 10-5).

FIGURE 10-6 Delta waves in Wolff-Parkinson White Syndrome

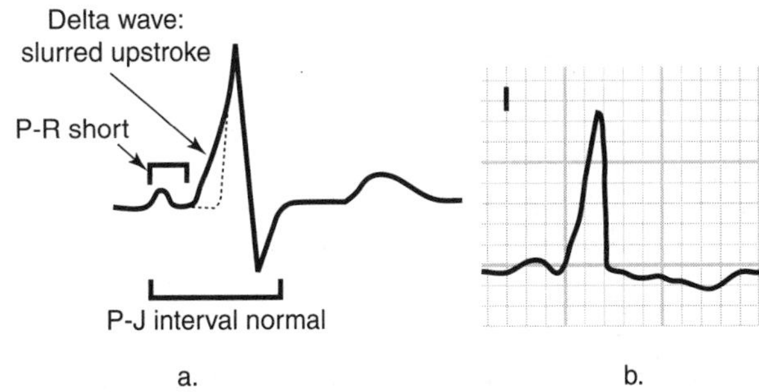

WOLFF-PARKINSON WHITE SYNDROME (WPW)

Often, patients presenting with WPW have a known history of this syndrome. WPW is caused by the presence of an accessory conduction pathway. The impulse traveling from the atria, instead of passing through the AV node, travels through another pathway, known as the Bundle of Kent. Since the AV node is bypassed, there is no mechanism to control the rate of impulses traveling to the ventricles, often resulting in a rapid ventricular response. The classic presentation on the ECG is the presence of delta wave—a notch or slurring of the front side of the QRS complex, and a shortened PR interval (<0.12 sec). See Figure 10-6.

Advanced Concepts with 12-Lead ECGs

The following are common causes of "false" ST segment elevation. These conditions can cause ST elevation not related to a cardiac event. The patient

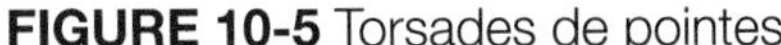

FIGURE 10-5 Torsades de pointes

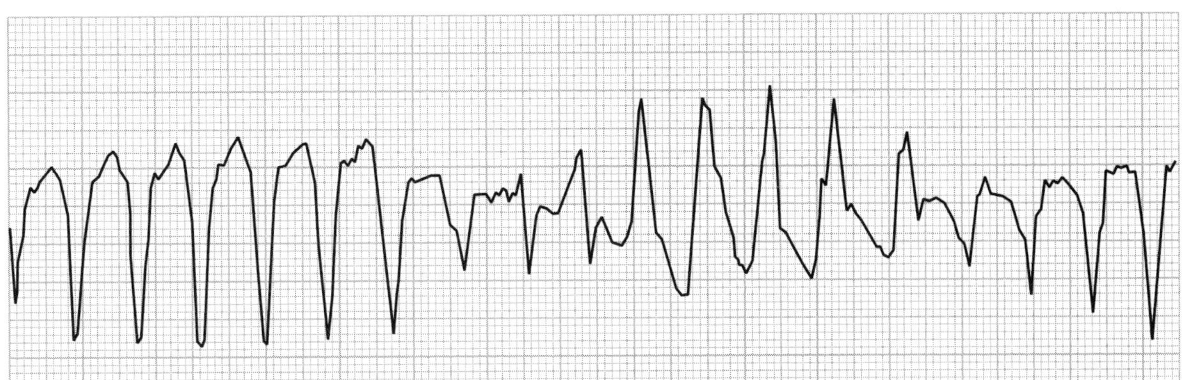

needs to be managed based on his symptoms and someone with expertise needs to evaluate the ECG.

1. Left bundle branch block—V1 will be wide (>0.12 sec) with a negative deflection.
2. Pacemaker—the QRS complex will be wide, pacemaker spikes may be visible.
3. Left ventricular hypertrophy—long (deep) QRS complexes usually in the V leads, T-wave in the opposite direction of the QRS.
4. Pericarditis—ST elevation in all leads. Pain less when patient sits forward; you may hear friction rub.
5. Early repolarization—elevation in lateral leads. Elevation is actually a gradual curve. Most common in young black males.
6. Hyperkalemia—high peaked T waves

There are common complications to expect with specific injured areas of the myocardium. Based on the patient's initial presentation, the clinician may find the ECG change initially and anticipate the potential complication or may find the complication first and then realize the cardiac-injured area after further evaluation.

1. V1-V2 injury pattern often damages the septum, bundle of HIS, and bundle branches; expect heart blocks and bundle branch blocks.
2. V3-V4 injury patterns damage the anterior left ventricle; expect heart blocks, bundle branch blocks, PVCs, left ventricular dysfunction, and CHF.
3. V5-V6, I, aVL injury patterns damage the high lateral wall of the left ventricle; expect heart blocks, left ventricular dysfunction and CHF.
4. Lead II, III, and aVF injury patterns may show injury to the inferior left ventricle, posterior left ventricle, or the right ventricle. Moving the V4 lead to the right chest and rerunning the 12-lead ECG looking specifically at V4 for elevation will help diagnose the right ventricular infarct. For a right infarct expect hypotension and severe hypotension if nitrates are administered. These patients require fluid boluses to increase preload. If the injury is truly in the left ventricle expect heart blocks, PACs, atrial fibrillation, and atrial flutter.
5. V1-V4 depression in all leads. While ECG depression is initially associated with ischemic changes, this unique pattern is often the sign of an infarction to the posterior wall of the left ventricle. Some may choose to place the V leads in the same location on the rear side of the chest to diagnose this infarction. Some may choose to utilize other tests such as cardiac enzymes or an echocardiogram. Others with expertise in interpreting 12-lead ECG will base the management of this patient on the clinical presentation and this specific ECG pattern. This patient may present with signs of left ventricular dysfunction. In either case the provider must recognize this patient may in fact be a candidate for acute reperfusion therapy despite the common ST elevation changes currently recommended.

Additional Pharmacologic Agents

There are a variety of medications available to the ACLS provider that are either not routinely used in resuscitation or stabilization scenarios, or are reserved for very specific situations.

Digibind

Classification:

Indications:

Digoxin toxicity (>10–15 ng/ml) with life-threatening arrhythmias, shock, hyperkalemia (>5 mEq/l)

Dosage:

Depends upon amount of Digoxin ingested (each 40 mg vial binds about 0.6 mg of digoxin).

Consideration:

Serum digoxin levels will rise after digibind therapy. Follow-up digoxin levels are not reliable indicators of need for continued digibind therapy.

Glucagon

Indication:

In ACLS, for treatment of toxic effects of beta blockers or calcium channel blockers.

Dosage:

3 mg IV/IO followed by infusion of 3 mg/hr as necessary

Considerations:

- Medication should be reconstituted with solution provided with dry dose.
- May cause hypoglycemia or vomiting.

Milrinone

Classification:

Indication:

- Congestive heart failure in post-open-heart surgery patients
- Shock without vasodilation
- Any case of myocardial dysfunction with increased pulmonary or systemic vascular resistance

Dosage:

- Load 50 µg/kg over 10 min
- Infuse 0.375–0.75 µg/kg/min for 2–3 days

Considerations:

- Shorter half-life than Inamrinone
- Patient should be monitored via PA catheter
- Reduce dose in impaired renal function
- Ensure adequate fluid volume; may cause hypotension in hypovolemic patients

Sotalol

Betapace

Classification:

Antiarrhythmic

Indications:

Ventricular and atrial arrhythmias

Dosage:

1–1.5 mg/kg body weight, then 10 mg/min IV

Considerations:

- IV form not yet approved in United States
- Has significant negative inotropic effects; should be infused slowly
- May cause bradycardia, hypotension, Torsades de pointes
- Reduce dose in patients with renal impairment

Ibutilide

Corvert

Classification:

Ibutilide

Indications:

- SVT
- Conversion of atrial fibrillation/flutter duration <48 hours

Dosage:

- 1 mg IV over 10 min; may repeat in 10 min if necessary
- May use weight-based dose 0.01 mg/kg if patient <60 kg

Considerations:

- Monitor patient for ventricular arrhythmias, specifically, Torsades de pointes
- Monitor ECG during administration and for 6 hr after

- Contraindicated in patients with QT interval >440 msec
- Patients with impaired left ventricular function are at highest risk of arrhythmias; keep defibrillator nearby

Inamrinone

Amrinone

Classification:

Phosphodiesterase enzyme inhibitor

Indication:

Severe CHF not responding to diuretics, other inotropic agents, or vasodilators

Dosage:

- Load 0.75 mg/kg over 2–3 min
- Follow with infusion 5–10 μg/kg/min titrated to effect

Considerations:

- Patient should be monitored via PA catheter
- Do not mix with dextrose solutions
- May cause tachycardia or hypotension
- Increased pumping increases myocardial oxygen demand and may cause myocardial ischemia
- Give loading dose more slowly (over 10–15 min) with poor left ventricular function

Isoproterenol

Isuprel

Classification:

Adrenergic stimulator (pure beta stimulator)

Indications:

Bradycardias refractory to atropine, pacing, dopamine, and epinephrine. (This drug rarely used due to its excessive increase in O_2 consumption.)

Dosage:

Mix 2 mg/500 cc D5W to yield 4 μg/cc. Infuse 2–10 μg/min (30–150 cc/hr) titrated to effective heart rate.

Route:

IV infusion only

Side effects:

Tachycardia, hypotension, ventricular ectopy, myocardial ischemia

Unique Arrest Situations

The following examples review management of patients suffering cardiovascular events from external causes. Many of these causes, though quite common, are not discussed in a standard ACLS course. These cases illustrate the need to have the ability to think outside the box in situations where the standard ACLS guidelines (i.e., a vasopressor and an antiarrhythmic) fail to resuscitate the patient.

While not every patient requires each management sequence and not all providers will have the ability or equipment to evaluate each condition, a standard evaluation, appropriate questioning, and a high index of suspicion for patients who fail to respond may mean the difference between a failed and a successful resuscitation. These are merely one option from the scientific guidelines and should not be construed as the only standard; other management is certainly acceptable.

Some interesting facts to keep in mind. The following will cause PEA as represented by the H's and T's throughout this book:

Hypoxia, hypovolemia, hypothermia, hyper/hypokalemia, hydrogen ion (acidosis) hypoglycemia, toxins (overdose), thromboemboli (pulmonary or coronary embolus), trauma-tension pneumothorax, tamponade (cardiac), too fast or too slow.

These situations will cause asystole:

Hypoxia, hypothermia, hypokalemia, hyperkalemia, acidosis, drug overdose, and death.

V-Fib or pulseless VT can be caused by anything.

Electrolyte Imbalances

Since not all providers have the ability to evaluate ABGs or blood work here are a few clues for patients not responding to your routine regime. Certainly the ability to rapidly obtain blood is best.

Renal Dialysis Patients

May have predialysis acidosis, hyperkalemia, hypoglycemia, or postdialysis hypokalemia and hypovolemia

Diabetics

May have acidosis, hypoglycemia, hypovolemia, hyperkalemia, hypokalemia

Alcoholics

May have hypokalemia, hypoglycemia, hypomagnesemia

Prolonged Vomiting

May have dehydration, metabolic acidosis, hypokalemia

Prolonged Diarrhea

May have dehydration, acidosis, hypokalemia, hypomagnesemia

Management of Electrolyte-Related Arrests Could Include:

Sodium bicarbonate for acidosis

Glucose check and dextrose for hypoglycemia

Calcium, glucose, bicarb for hyperkalemia

Potassium replacement for hypokalemia

Consider thiamine for alcoholics

Magnesium sulfate for potential hypomagnesaemia (often Torsades de pointes)

Unique Respiratory Conditions

COPD and asthma have caused arrests in the old and the young from respiratory failure and acidosis. There have also been numerous cases of tension pneumothoraxes developing.

- Pneumothorax patients may require pleural decompression if they fail to respond to standard ACLS or have poor BVM compliance and diminished lung sounds.

Drowning

- Hypoxia and acidosis are the initial causes.
- Consider C-spine management, sodium bicarbonate, and hypothermia.
- Hypothermia—handle gently, increase temperature, and begin ACLS slowly.

Trauma Arrests

- Though survivability rates are low, scene management should include spinal immobilization, airway control, bleeding control, and a rapid search for reversible conditions such as tension pneumothorax, and V-fib. IV fluids and medication should take place en route to a trauma facility. Some areas may choose not to resuscitate significant trauma.

Pregnancy

- Shift fetus to the left.
- Consider C-section if there is no response to 5 minutes of ACLS.
- Do not change the standard ACLS protocols.

Anaphylaxis

- Allergic reactions, while usually easily reversible, may progress to cardiovascular collapse due to profound vasodilation and hypoperfusion.
- For patients in near arrest or arrest states, administer epinephrine IV rather than sq., then follow standard ACLS to manage arrhythmias. Emphasis should be placed on securing an appropriate airway.

Arrests Related to Overdose

The initial management for drug-induced arrests is basically unchanged. The following outlines consideration in specific overdoses:

Cocaine Tachyarrhythmias, vasoconstriction, pulmonary edema, and seizures.

- **SVT** Often short-lived, not requiring therapy. However, for sustained SVT consider using a benzodiazepine such as Diazepam in a dose of 5–20 mg IV over 5–20 minutes.
- **Hemodynamically stable VT** Consider benzodiazepines such as Diazepam 5–20 mg IV over 5–20 min. If persistent, try lidocaine 1–1.5 mg/kg IV (watch for toxicity due to synergistic toxic effects in the presence of cocaine). Follow with sodium bicarbonate 1–2 mEq/kg IV.
- **Ventricular fib** Defibrillate, follow with epinephrine 1 mg IV, limited to single dose or repeated in 5–10 min, or Vasopressin 40 u IV × 1. Follow with lidocaine 1–1.5 mg/kg IV, and if VF persists, follow with sodium bicarbonate 1–2 mEq/kg.
- **Hypertension** Treat initially with benzodiazepine. Follow with vasodilator such as nitroglycerine or Nitroprusside (nitroglycerine preferred if concurrent chest pain).
- **Do not use beta blockers** Blocking beta stimulus may allow the alpha properties of cocaine to continue unopposed, potentially increasing blood pressure. A pure alpha-blocker such as phentolamine (1 mg q2–3 min up to 10 mg) may be used.
- **Pulmonary edema** Standard medical management including positive pressure ventilation
- **Acute coronary syndromes** With cocaine use, more often due to spasm rather than thrombus. Use O_2, ASA, NTG, titrated doses of benzodiazepine. No beta blockers. May utilize magnesium and morphine.

Tricyclic Antidepressants Cardiotoxic when overdosed. Expect mental status changes, tachycardias, prolonged QT intervals, and anticholinergic effects. Interventions include:

- Activated charcoal within 1 hr of ingestion
- Gastric lavage for unconscious patients
- If seizures occur, terminate immediately with benzodiazepines
- Alkalinization with sodium bicarb if:
  - QRS > 100 ms
  - Ventricular arrhythmias
  - Hypotension unresponsive to saline bolus of 500–1000 cc
- Magnesium if prolonged QT interval or Torsades
- If cardiac arrest: Most often PEA
  - In addition to PEA interventions, add hyperventilation, early fluid-NS at 1000 cc/hr, Sodium Bicarb 1–2 mEq/kg IVP, Bicarb infusion

Digitalis Overdose may cause bradyarrhythmias and heart failure, ventricular arrhythmias, and hyperkalemia. Treatment should include:

- Replacing sodium, potassium, and volume
- Activated charcoal within 1 hour of ingestion
- Highly selective use of transvenous pacemakers due to frequency of pacemaker induced arrhythmias
- Atropine for symptomatic bradycardias
- Fab fragment therapy (Digibind) if:
  - Life-threatening arrhythmias refractory to other therapy
  - Shock or CHF
  - K+ >5 mEq/L
  - Serum Dig levels >10–15 in adults
  - Cardiac arrest
  - Acute ingestion >10 mg
- Potassium, magnesium, and saline for arrhythmias
- Lidocaine IVP if arrhythmias do not respond to K+ magnesium, and saline
- Phenytoin may be used in place of lidocaine

- If VF, use VF algorithm but add Mg 1–2 g following lidocaine, then Fab fragment antibodies
- Defibrillate q60 sec

Calcium Channel Blocker and Beta Blocker Toxicity May cause hypotension, decreased contractility, bradycardias, decreased LOC, seizures, hypoglycemia and hyperkalemia with beta blockers, hyperglycemia with calcium channel blockers, rapid progression to shock. Treatment should include:

- O_2, ECG, monitor BP, establish vascular access
- Volume for hypotension
- Check blood glucose
- Activated charcoal within 1 hour of ingestion with mild hemodynamic effects
- Rapid sequence intubation and gastric lavage for severe hemodynamic toxicity
- For calcium channel blocker overdose, to treat myocardial dysfunction:
  - NS boluses 500–1000 cc
  - Epinephrine infusion 2–10 μg/min
  - Calcium chloride if shock refractory to fluids and epinephrine
  - Pacing for bradycardia
- For beta blocker overdose, to treat myocardial dysfunction:
  - NS boluses
  - Vasopressor infusion (epinephrine, norepinephrine, dobutamine, dopamine)
  - Glucagon 1–5 mg IV
  - Isoproterinol

Narcotics or Benzodiazepines Generally cause respiratory arrest

- For narcotics, Narcan 2 mg up to 10 mg
- For benzodiazepines, Romazicon 0.2 mg slowly up to 1 mg

CHAPTER 11

Practice Tests

Tips for the Written Exam

The standardized exam is the same type most of us are used to taking since gradeschool. A question, scenario, or problem is presented, then the student is given a choice of four possible options. Generally one choice has nothing to do with the correct answer, one is "in the ball park," and two are potentials. If you can rule out the obviously wrong answers, then look for clues such as two of the answers that mean the same thing or have nothing to do with one another, your chance of figuring out the correct answer for those you are unfamiliar with is much greater. However, there is no substitute for actually being familiar with the information enough that you can recall the correct answer when asked.

These tips for reducing stress will increase your effectiveness before the program:

- Prepare. Read the information, take the pretest, study a bit for a week or two before the class.
- Focus on your "problem areas" early on but do not forget to review all information.
- Eat healthy meals for several days before the exam to give you "brain energy."
- Show up on time; don't create stress for yourself by being late for the program or possibly getting lost.
- If you are one of those people who gets cold in large rooms, bring a jacket.

Taking the exam:

- Read the *entire* question; ask yourself what do they want to know?
- Read *all* options; often A is a good choice but C or D is a better choice.
- Remember you are testing on the *course material,* not necessarily what you do in real life.
- Look specifically at what *you are being asked;* do not "read into the question."
- If you do not know an answer, skip it and come back to it later; something may trigger recall.
- If there is more than one possible answer, choose the *best* option (not, "well it could be...")
- If any part of the answer is incorrect, the entire answer is wrong (i.e., correct med, wrong dose).
- RELAX. If you have taken the time to prepare and review these pretests, you will be familiar with all the standard ACLS information.

ACLS Practice Exam 1

1. The following patients presented to the emergency department with signs and symptoms of a stroke. Noncontrast CT is negative for hemorrhage. Which have no contraindications for fibrinolytic therapy for stroke treatment?
   A. A 65-year-old woman who underwent colon resection 3 days ago
   B. A 76-year-old man whose symptoms began 4½ hours ago
   C. A pregnant 40-year-old woman with a blood pressure of 122/74 whose symptoms began 2 hours ago
   D. An 80-year-old woman with blood pressure of 140/96 whose symptoms began 2 hours ago

2. Which of the following is not an indication for transcutaneous pacing?
   A. Witnessed asystole
   B. Second-degree (2°) type II AV block with hypotension and dizziness
   C. Sinus bradycardia with blood pressure 74/50
   D. Third-degree (3°) heart block with decreased level of consciousness

3. What is the appropriate dose of Amiodarone for the awake patient with ventricular tachycardia, no chest pain, clear lungs, and a blood pressure of 110/66?
   A. 300 mg in 50 cc NS over 10 minutes
   B. 150 mg IV
   C. 300 mg IV
   D. 450 mg in 250 cc at 33 cc/hr

4. Which of the following is true about end tidal CO_2 measurement following endotracheal intubation?
   A. False positive readings can be obtained following intubation of the esophagus.
   B. Failure to detect CO_2 is not a definitive sign of improper ET tube placement.
   C. CO_2 detection is one piece of information that can assist in confirming proper tube placement.
   D. All of the above

5. An employee at a golf course complains of chest pain and then becomes unresponsive. His coworkers call 911 and retrieve an AED from the clubhouse. Following analysis, the AED states "no shock advised." What is the next appropriate step for the rescuers?
   A. Check for breathing and a pulse. If indicated, begin compressions and ventilations.
   B. Check the pads to be sure they have adhered well to the chest.

C. Push the analyze button again.
D. Turn off the AED and proceed with chest compressions and ventilations.

6. For which of the patients in PEA (pulseless electrical activity) is atropine indicated?
   A. A 60-year-old woman with a history of GI bleed and sinus tachycardia, rate 110 on the monitor.
   B. A patient found unresponsive with sinus bradycardia, rate 44 on the monitor.
   C. A dehydrated patient with poor skin turgor and normal sinus rhythm, rate 88 on the monitor.
   D. A patient who has overdosed on Valium with accelerated junctional rhythm, rate 66 on the monitor.

7. What is the appropriate dose of sodium bicarbonate for the 80-kg patient in cardiac arrest?
   A. 40 mEq IV followed by a repeat dose of 80 mEq if necessary.
   B. 80 mEq IV followed by a repeat dose of 80 mEq if necessary.
   C. 40 mEq IV followed by a repeat dose of 40 mEq if necessary.
   D. 80 mEq IV followed by a repeat dose of 40 mEq if necessary.

8. What should be done immediately prior to discharging defibrillator?
   A. State "clear" and visually scan the area.
   B. Charge the paddles and ensure that the "synch" button is not pushed.
   C. Apply conductive gel to the defibrillator paddles.
   D. Turn off the monitor to avoid electrical damage when the patient is shocked.

9. Which of the following agents is indicated for a 50-year-old man complaining of chest pain unrelieved by nitroglycerine with ST elevation in three related ECG leads?
   A. Heparin
   B. Morphine
   C. Epinephrine
   D. Procainamide

10. Which of the following patients presenting with acute myocardial infarction is most likely to present with vague or unusual symptoms?
    A. A 45-year-old woman with a history of stroke.
    B. A 72-year-old man with no history of heart disease.
    C. A 70-year-old man in the intensive care unit following radical prostatectomy.
    D. A 70-year-old woman with a 10-year history of adult onset diabetes.

11. Which of the following parameters would not be assessed to determine if a patient is symptomatic from an arrhythmia?
    A. Symmetry of motor strength.
    B. Mental status.
    C. Blood pressure.
    D. Presence or absence of chest pain.

12. Which is the appropriate dose of IV push lidocaine for the 90-kg patient in ventricular fibrillation?
    A. 135 mg.
    B. 125 mg.
    C. 75 mg.
    D. 45 mg.

13. Which is the proper sequence for performing synchronized cardioversion?
    A. Avoid sedation until the patient is stable, press the synch button, confirm visual cues that monitor is in "synch," select the highest energy level, position

pads or paddles, press charge button, discharge paddles.

B. Consider sedation, turn on monitor, press the synch button, confirm visual cues that monitor is in "synch," disconnect electrodes to avoid damage to the monitor, select appropriate energy, position pads or paddles, press charge button, clear patient, discharge paddles.

C. Consider sedation, turn on monitor and attach leads to patient, press the synch button, confirm visual cues that monitor is in "synch," select appropriate energy, position pads or paddles, press charge button, clear patient, discharge paddles.

D. Consider sedation, turn off monitor and attach leads to patient, press the synch button, confirm visual cues that monitor is not in "synch," select the highest energy, position pads or paddles, press charge button, clear patient, discharge paddles.

14. Your 60-year-old patient admitted to the hospital presses his call button and tells you that he had pressure in the center of his chest, rated 9 on a scale of 0 to 10. His vital signs are as follows: HR 110/min, resp 14/min, BP 132/86, O_2 saturation 96%. He is visibly uncomfortable, diaphoretic, and nauseated. Which of the following may be included in his plan of care for the next 20 minutes?

A. Oxygen, nitroglycerine, 12-lead ECG if pain not relieved, aspirin.

B. Oxygen, nitroglycerine ×3, aspirin, 12-lead ECG, ACE inhibitors.

C. Oxygen, nitroglycerine, aspirin, morphine if nitroglycerine ×3 fails to relieve the pain.

D. Oxygen, nitroglycerine, aspirin, fibrinolytics if 12-lead ECG negative for injury.

15. You receive a patient in your intensive care unit from the emergency department postventricular fibrillation, with successful resuscitation. The patient has two large antecubital IVs with dopamine and lidocaine hanging, is being ventilated via an endotracheal tube inserted in the ED, and shows sinus tachycardia on the monitor. After transfer to the bed, you begin assessment, and upon checking blood pressure, you discover the patient has no pulse. You call for help and begin chest compressions. Your compressions produce a strong pulse, but there continues to be no pulse when compressions are stopped and the monitor continues to show sinus tach. What is the next most appropriate action?

A. Administer epinephrine 3 mg IV.

B. Assess endotracheal tube placement and breath sounds.

C. Draw blood for arterial blood gas.

D. Send blood sample for electrolyte and cardiac enzymes.

16. A 79-year-old woman collapses at home and her family calls 911. Paramedics arrive within 3 minutes and find the woman pulseless and apneic. They begin CPR and attach the cardiac monitor, which shows ventricular fibrillation. Which is the most appropriate next action?

A. Defibrillate immediately and secure an advanced airway.

B. Deliver a precordial thump, and resume CPR if the rhythm does not change.

C. Continue CPR for a total of 2 minutes, recheck the rhythm, and defibrillate at 360 joules if VF persists.

D. Establish venous access, preferably in the antecubital space, administer 40 u of vasopressin IV, and defibrillate after 1 minute of CPR.

17. A 70-kg patient in cardiac arrest converts from VF to sinus rhythm at 70 bpm. He

remains pulseless. The resuscitation team continues CPR, reconfirms that the tracheal tube is properly placed, with ventilation producing bilateral breath sounds and chest rise. The last medication administered (prior to rhythm change) was lidocaine 100 mg 4 minutes ago. Which of the following medications is most appropriate to give next?

A. Atropine 1.0 mg IVP.
B. Epinephrine 1.0 mg IVP.
C. Lidocaine 100 mg IVP.
D. Sodium bicarbonate 100 mEq IVP.

18. A patient has just been intubated following severe respiratory distress. Which of the following is true about confirming endotracheal tube placement?

A. If the patient has bilateral breath sounds on auscultation, no further confirmation is necessary.
B. Confirmation procedures such as CO_2 detection should occur as soon as possible.
C. Chest X ray to confirm tube placement should be performed as soon as possible.
D. CO_2 detection is not a reliable indicator of tube placement in perfusing patients.

19. Which of the following actions is not necessary prior to defibrillation?

A. Disconnect the bag valve mask from the endotracheal tube and step away from the patient.
B. Check the scene to be sure no one is touching the patient.
C. Confirm that the rhythm on the monitor is ventricular fibrillation or pulseless ventricular tachycardia.
D. Turn off IV pumps so they will not be damaged by the electrical shock.

20. A patient who has called you to her bedside because she feels palpitations has a heart rate of 190 bpm, with a narrow complex tachycardia on the monitor. Which of the following statements displays an indication for synchronized cardioversion?

A. The patient says, "Whew! It feels like my heart is beating really fast!"
B. The nursing assistant says, "The patient's blood pressure is 120/66."
C. The monitor tech says, "This patient's rhythm one hour ago was atrial flutter with a ventricular response of 80."
D. The respiratory therapist says, "The patient has rales bilaterally, oxygen saturation (SaO_2) has dropped to 90%, and her blood pressure is now 80/50."

21. An awake alert 50-kg patient with SVT on her monitor has a BP of 150/80 and HR 185 bpm. She denies chest pain, her lungs are clear, and vagal maneuvers fail to slow her heart rate. Which of the following interventions is most appropriate?

A. Sedate and cardiovert at 100 joules.
B. Administer Diltiazem 35 mg IVP.
C. Administer lidocaine 50 mg IVP.
D. Administer adenosine 6 mg IVP.

22. Endotracheal intubation has just been performed on a 70-year-old male in cardiac arrest. Upon auscultation, you note no sounds over the epigastrium, audible breath sounds over the right lung fields, and no breath sounds over left lung fields. What is the most likely explanation for these findings?

A. The tube was advanced too far and passed into the right main stem bronchus.
B. The tube was not advanced far enough and is in the hypoharynx.
C. The tube was mistakenly placed in the esophagus.
D. The patient has a right tension pneumothorax.

23. Which of the following is true about the use of Vasopressin during cardiac arrest?
    A. Administer vasopressin 40 u IV to enhance myocardial contractility.
    B. Administer vasopressin 40 u IV in place of the first or second dose of epinephrine, if desired.
    C. Administer vasopressin 40 u IV q3–5 minutes in cardiac arrest.
    D. Administer vasopressin 40 u IV in place of lidocaine to decrease myocardial irritability in ventricular fibrillation.

24. Which of the following is true about ventricular fibrillation?
    A. Ventricular fibrillation should always be treated with immediate defibrillation.
    B. Ventricular fibrillation causes a 50% drop in stroke volume.
    C. Ventricular fibrillation responds well to early IV administration of adenosine.
    D. Ventricular fibrillation does not produce a palpable pulse.

25. Which action is recommended to open the airway of a 55-year-old pulseless, apneic victim found unresponsive in his hospital bed?
    A. Jaw thrust with cervical spine stabilization.
    B. Insertion of a nasal pharyngeal airway (NPA).
    C. Tongue jaw lift.
    D. Head tilt–chin lift.

ACLS Practice Exam 2

1. A patient in cardiac arrest has been intubated with a #7.5 cuffed tracheal tube. Tube placement has been confirmed via visualization, auscultation, and use of a colormetric CO_2 detector device. CPR is in progress. Which of the following statements best describes the ventilations and compressions that should be provided?
    A. Alternate 15 compressions and 2 ventilations.
    B. Provide continuous compressions at a rate of about 80 per minute, without pausing for ventilations, and rescue breaths at a rate of 1 every 5 seconds, without pausing for compressions.
    C. Alternate 30 compressions and 2 ventilations.
    D. Provide continuous compressions at a rate of 100 per minute, without pausing for ventilations and rescue breaths at a rate of 1 every 6–7 seconds, without pausing for compressions.

2. You are providing bag valve mask (BVM) ventilations to a patient in respiratory arrest. Which of the following is true about ventilating with a BVM attached to an oxygen source?
    A. Ventilations should be slow; deliver each breath over 2–3 seconds.
    B. Ventilations should be rapid; ventilate at least once every 5 seconds.
    C. Ventilation with a bag valve mask requires skill and practice and should not be performed by someone who is not properly trained.
    D. Ventilation with a bag valve mask, if properly performed, can deliver between 60 and 70% oxygen to the patient.

3. Endotracheal intubation has been performed for a patient in cardiopulmonary arrest. Bilateral breath sounds are auscultated, the chest is rising with each ventilation, but your end tidal CO_2 detector

fails to detect exhaled CO_2. What is the most likely explanation of this finding?

A. The CO_2 detector device is faulty and should be replaced with a new one.

B. Poor pulmonary blood flow in cardiac arrest often fails to produce measurable amounts of exhaled CO_2.

C. The tracheal tube has erroneously been placed in the esophagus.

D. The patient is not being oxygenated well enough to produce CO_2 and should be ventilated more rapidly.

4. A 160-lb patient in ventricular fibrillation (VF) has failed to respond to a defibrillatory shock at 360 joules, and VF persists. Team members perform endotracheal intubation, confirm tube placement, secure the tracheal tube, and insert an 18 gauge IV catheter in the antecubital space. Which of the following medications should be given first?

A. Atropine 1.0 mg IV.

B. Epinephrine 1.0 mg IV.

C. Lidocaine 100 mg IV.

D. Sodium bicarbonate 100 mEq IV.

5. A patient is found unresponsive, apneic, and pulseless. The resuscitation team begins CPR and attaches the cardiac monitor, which displays sinus tachycardia with a heart rate of 116 bpm. Which sequence of treatment recommendations (algorithm) should you follow?

A. Asystole.

B. Unstable tachycardia.

C. Ventricular fibrillation.

D. Pulseless electrical activity.

6. Which of the following steps should you take to confirm that the flat line seen on a cardiac monitor is true asystole?

A. Turn the monitor off and on again.

B. Turn the monitor gain up.

C. Check cable to be sure they are disconnected.

D. Turn the lead select from lead II to paddles and back.

7. Which is the most appropriate way to reverse respiratory acidosis in the cardiac arrest patient?

A. Hyperventilate with 100% oxygen at a rate of 18–20 per minute.

B. Administer a 300 cc fluid bolus.

C. Administer sodium bicarbonate 1.0 mEq/kg.

D. Ventilate with 100% oxygen at a rate of 8–10 per minute.

8. Which of the following is a rapidly reversible cause of prehospital asystole?

A. Pulmonary embolus.

B. Serum potassium of 7.2 mEq/dl.

C. Core body temperature 87°F.

D. Opiate overdose.

9. A 79-year-old woman collapses at home and her family calls 911. Paramedics arrive within 3 minutes and find the woman pulseless and apneic. They begin CPR and attach the cardiac monitor, which shows ventricular fibrillation. Which is the most appropriate next action?

A. Defibrillate immediately and secure an advanced airway.

B. Deliver a precordial thump, and resume CPR if the rhythm does not change.

C. Continue CPR for a total of 2 minutes, recheck the rhythm, and defibrillate at 360 joules if VF persists.

D. Establish venous access, preferably in the antecubital space, administer 40 u of Vasopressin IV and defibrillate after 1 minute of CPR.

10. After one defibrillatory shock, an 80-kg patient in cardiac arrest converts from VF to sinus rhythm at 70 bpm. He remains pulseless. The resuscitation team continues CPR, reconfirms that the tracheal tube is properly placed, with ventilation producing bilateral breath sounds and chest rise. The last medication administered (prior to rhythm change) was amiodarone 300 mg IV 4 minutes ago. Which of the following medications is most appropriate to give next?
    A. Atropine 1.0 mg IVP.
    B. Vasopressin 40 u IVP.
    C. Lidocaine 100 mg IVP.
    D. Sodium bicarbonate 100 mEq IVP.

11. A 60-year-old woman is leaning to the right and has slurred speech. You suspect stroke. Before sending her to CT scan, you should rule out which non-stroke causes of these findings?
    A. Hypertension.
    B. Hypoglycemia.
    C. Hyperkalemia.
    D. Use of stimulant medications.

12. Which of the following actions is true about defibrillation?
    A. When using hands-free pads it is not necessary to call "clear" before shocking.
    B. If compressing prior to defibrillation, be sure to stop compressions for at least 10 seconds to allow the defibrillator to charge and everyone to clear the patient.
    C. Turn off IV pumps so they will not be damaged by the electrical shock.
    D. Following defibrillation, immediately resume CPR beginning with compressions.

13. Which of the following best describes the use of the bag valve mask (BVM) device to ventilate a nonbreathing patient?
    A. The use of the device is simple and requires minimal training and practice.
    B. The bag should be squeezed gently over approximately 1 second.
    C. The contents of the bag should be completely delivered to maximize tidal volume.
    D. It is not necessary to use an oral pharyngeal airway (OPA) with BVM if the head tilt–chin lift is appropriately maintained.

14. A 60-year-old woman is found unresponsive, with a thready pulse, a heart rate of 180, and ventricular tachycardia on the monitor. Her BP is 74/40, RR 10/min, her skin is cool, and her periphery is pale. You would most accurately describe her status as:
    A. Acute coronary syndrome.
    B. Unstable tachycardia.
    C. Severe hypovolemic hypotension.
    D. Stable tachycardia.

15. What is the most appropriate next set of interventions?
    A. Administer oxygen and synchronize cardiovert.
    B. Obtain central venous access and administer lidocaine 1.5 mg IVP.
    C. Administer nasal cannula oxygen and prepare for overdrive pacing.
    D. Insert a peripheral IV, obtain a 12-lead ECG, administer sedation, and prepare to defibrillate.

16. Which of the following will interfere with an AED's ability to accurately analyze a patient's cardiac rhythm?
    A. Chest compressions.
    B. Patient movement.

C. Bag valve mask ventilation.
D. All of the above.

17. If an AED is available at the scene of a witnessed cardiac arrest, when should it be applied to the victim?
A. As soon as it is available.
B. After it is established that the patient is not breathing.
C. After two slow rescue breaths have been delivered.
D. After is established that the patient is pulseless.

18. Which of the following is true about placement for AEDs, transcutaneous pacing, or hands-free defibrillation or cardioversion?
A. Extra conductive medium should be placed on the chest prior to pad placement.
B. Pads stick well to oily or diaphoretic skin.
C. Pads may be placed over implanted devices or bone.
D. Hair in the area where pads will be placed should be removed if possible.

19. Which of the following describes a hazard that should be addressed prior to delivering a shock with an AED?
A. The patient is laying on a metal grate.
B. The patient's wife is holding his hand.
C. The patient is laying in a puddle of water.
D. All of the above.

20. What should the rescuer do if, following rhythm analysis, an AED delivers a "no shock advised" message?
A. Turn the patient to the recovery position and continue to observe.
B. Turn off the AED and restart.
C. Begin ventilations with a bag valve mask 10 times per minute.
D. Check ABCs and begin CPR if the patient is pulseless and apneic.

21. Which action is recommended to open the airway of a 55-year-old pulseless, apneic victim found face down on the floor beside his hospital bed?
A. Jaw thrust with cervical spine stabilization.
B. Insertion of a nasal pharyngeal airway (NPA).
C. Tongue jaw lift.
D. Head tilt–chin lift.

22. If an AED is available at the scene of an unwitnessed cardiac arrest with suspected long down time, when should it be applied to the victim?
A. As soon as it is available.
B. After it is established that the patient is not breathing.
C. After two slow rescue breaths have been delivered.
D. During CPR, with analysis following 2 minutes of CPR.

23. A patient is found unresponsive, apneic, and pulseless. The resuscitation team begins CPR and attaches the cardiac monitor, which displays sinus tachycardia with a heart rate of 116 bpm. Which sequence of treatment recommendations (algorithm) should you follow?
A. Asystole.
B. Unstable tachycardia.
C. Ventricular fibrillation.
D. Pulseless electrical activity.

24. How much epinephrine should be administered to the patient in asystole?
    A. 10 mg of a 1:10,000 solution.
    B. 3 mg of a 1:1,000 solution.
    C. 3 cc of a 1:10,000 solution.
    D. 10 cc of a 1:10,000 solution.

25. What is the appropriate dose of amiodarone for an awake patient in ventricular tachycardia with clear lungs, BP 108/60 and RR 12 SaO_2 97%?
    A. 150 mg.
    B. 1 mg/kg.
    C. 300 mg.
    D. .04 mg/kg.

Answer Keys

ANSWER KEY CHAPTER 2—AIRWAY MANAGEMENT

1. b
2. c
3. a
4. c
5. a
6. b
7. c
8. a
9. a
10. c
11. d
12. c
13. d
14. a
15. b
16. c
17. a
18. d
19. b
20. b

ANSWER KEY CHAPTER 3—ECG PRACTICE TEST 1

1. Ventricular pacemaker with intermittent capture
2. Sinus bradycardia with unifocal PVCs
3. Atrial fibrillation with a ventricular response of 90
4. Supraventricular tachycardia
5. Sinus bradycardia
6. Second-degree AV block, type II
7. Ventricular tachycardia
8. Normal sinus rhythm with unifocal PVCs
9. Asystole
10. Atrial flutter with ventricular response 7011; ventricular tachycardia
12. Ventricular fibrillation
13. Second-degree AV block type I
14. Idioventricular rhythm
15. Second-degree AV block, type II
16. Supraventricular tachycardia
17. Junctional rhythm
18. Third-degree heart block
19. Ventricular fibrillation
20. Normal sinus rhythm
21. Normal sinus rhythm
22. Ventricular tachycardia
23. Third-degree heart block
24. Atrial flutter
25. Functional rhythm
26. Ventricular tachycardia
27. Atrial fibrillation
28. Ventricular fibrillation
29. Atrial tachycardia (SVT)
30. Ventricular pacing with 100% capture

31. Normal sinus rhythm
32. Atrial fibrillation
33. Second-degree heart block Type I
34. Sinus rhythm with PVCs
35. Junctional rhythm
36. Sinus bradycardia with first-degree AV block
37. Sinus rhythm with unifocal PVCs
38. Ventricular tachycardia
39. Sinus tachycardia
40. Sinus rhythm with first-degree AV block
41. Sinus rhythm with first-degree AV block
42. Atrial tachycardia
43. Third-degree heart block
44. Third-degree heart block
45. Sinus bradycardia
46. Junctional rhythm
47. Second-degree heart block type II
48. Sinus tachycardia
49. Atrial fibrillation with PVCs
50. Atrial flutter

ANSWER KEY CHAPTER 3—ECG PRACTICE TEST 2

1. Accelerated junctional rhythm
2. Atrial flutter
3. Atrial tachycardia
4. Second-degree heart block Type I
5. Ventricular tachycardia
6. Ventricular pacing with 100% capture
7. Ventricular fibrillation
8. Second-degree heart block Type II
9. Sinus bradycardia
10. Atrial tachycardia
11. Idioventricular rhythm
12. Atrial fibrillation
13. Sinus tachycardia
14. Sinus rhythm with PVCs
15. Idioventricular rhythm
16. Accelerated junctional rhythm
17. Ventricular fibrillation
18. Atrial flutter
19. Junctional tachycardia
20. Sinus tachycardia
21. Normal sinus rhythm
22. Ventricular tachycardia → Ventricular fibrillation
23. Second-degree heart block Type II
24. Idioventricular rhythm
25. Second-degree heart block Type I
26. Atrial flutter
27. Atrial flutter
28. Second-degree heart block Type I
29. Ventricular fibrillation
30. Sinus tachycardia
31. Idioventricular rhythm
32. Ventricular fibrillation
33. Sinus bradycardia
34. Second-degree heart block Type II
35. Supraventricular tachycardia
36. First-degree heart block
37. Atrial fibrillation
38. Sinus tachycardia
39. Ventricular tachycardia
40. Third-degree heart block
41. Ventricular pacing with +sensing and 100% capture
42. Normal sinus rhythm
43. Second-degree heart block Type I
44. Sinus bradycardia
45. Second-degree heart block Type II
46. Second-degree heart block Type I
47. Supraventricular tachycardia
48. Third-degree heart block
49. Ventricular pacing with 100% capture
50. Ventricular tachycardia

ANSWER KEY: CHAPTER 4—12-LEAD ECGs

1. ST elevation in V1, V2, V3, V4 = AMI—Injury to the anterior and lateral portion.
2. Normal 12-lead ECG. No significant ST depression, inversions, or elevations.
3. Inverted T-waves, ST depression lead II, III, aVF = ischemia in the inferior portion.
4. ST elevation lead II, III, aVF = AMI—injury to the inferior portion with ST depression in V2, V3, lead I, and aVL = ischemia in the anterior portion.

5. ST elevation leads I, aVL, V1, V2, V3 = AMI—injury to the anterior and septal portion with ST depression lead II, III, aVF = ischemia to the inferior portion.

ANSWER KEY: CHAPTER 6—PHARMACOLOGY OVERVIEW

1. g
2. l
3. e
4. s
5. a
6. j
7. p
8. t
9. b
10. c
11. r
12. h
13. d
14. n
15. i
16. q
17. k
18. f
19. o
20. m
21. 0.5–1.0 mg IV
22. 6 mg IV
23. 40 u IV
24. 0.5–1.0 mg/kg IV
25. 2–4 lpm via nasal cannula
26. 300 mg IV
27. 1.0 mg IV
28. 1.0 mg/kg IV
29. 3 mg or 0.04 mg/kg IV
30. 20–50 mg/min IV
31. 162–325 mg po
32. 2–4 mg/min
33. 150 mg
34. 3.0 mg/kg
35. 2–4 mg IV (may repeat)
36. 1.0 mg
37. 0.3–0.4 mg sl may repeat q5 min
38. 90–100% (15 l on flowmeter)
39. 5–10 μg/kg/min
40. 2–2.5 mg IV
41. b
42. c
43. d
44. a
45. d

ANSWER KEY : CHAPTER 7—STROKE PRACTICE TEST 1

1. c
2. e
3. c
4. b
5. c
6. a
7. d
8. c
9. b
10. e

ANSWER KEY: CHAPTER 7—STROKE PRACTICE TEST 2

1. b
2. d
3. f
4. d
5. a
6. a
7. b
8. a
9. b
10. d

ANSWER KEY: CHAPTER 8—ACUTE CORONARY SYNDROMES

1. b
2. a
3. c
4. b
5. d

6. c
7. c
8. b
9. d
10. a

ANSWER KEY: CHAPTER 11—ACLS PRACTICE EXAM 1

1. d
2. a
3. b
4. d
5. a
6. b
7. d
8. a
9. b
10. d
11. a
12. a
13. c
14. c
15. b
16. c
17. b
18. b
19. d
20. d
21. d
22. a
23. b
24. d
25. d

ANSWER KEY: CHAPTER 11—ACLS PRACTICE EXAM 2

1. d
2. c
3. b
4. b
5. d
6. b
7. d
8. d
9. c
10. b
11. b
12. d
13. b
14. b
15. a
16. d
17. d
18. d
19. d
20. d
21. a
22. d
23. d
24. d
25. a

Glossary

ACLS Advanced cardiac life support

ACS (Acute coronary syndrome) A range of cardiac conditions involving decreased oxygen delivery to myocardial tissue. Includes myocardial ischemia, angina, unstable angina, and acute myocardial infarction

Bolus IV push, or administration of moderate or high volume of fluid over a relatively short period of time

Cardiac output The amount of blood ejected from the left ventricle in 1 minute. Expressed by the equation: Cardiac output = Heart rate × stroke volume

Chronotropic effect Pharmacologic effect causing increase in heart rate

Combitube (Esophageal Tracheal Combitube) A dual lumen airway tube ideally inserted into the esophagus. The tube has a port in each lumen to facilitate ventilation from either port, as needed.

Ejection fraction The percentage of blood in the ventricle that is ejected each time the ventricle contracts.

Hypothermia Low body temperature. For ACLS, defined as core body temperature <94°F

Inotropic effect Pharmacologic effect causing increase in force of contraction of the ventricle

Infarction Death of tissue. In the case of myocardial infarction, due to lack of oxygen, most often occlusion of coronary artery.

IO (Intraosseous) An alternative route for administration of medications and fluids when intravenous access is not available

Ischemia A state of low oxygenation in myocardial cells

LMA (Laryngeal mask airway) A noninvasive airway, used as a BLS airway device, when intubation is delayed or not possible; occludes the supraglottic area and facilitates oxygen flow to the trachea

PCI (Percutaneous cardiac intervention) Invasive cardiac procedures, such as angioplasty or stenting

Perfusion Delivery of oxygenated blood to tissues

Perfusing A state where oxygenated blood is delivered to tissues (i.e., a patient with a pulse)

Stroke volume The amount of blood ejected from the ventricle in one contraction

Tidal volume The amount of air taken into the lungs in one breath or ventilation

Vasopressor Medication that causes vascular constriction

Index

A

B

P

Q

R

T